Creative Approaches to Health and Social Care Education

Creative Approaches to Health and Social Care Education

Knowing Me, Understanding You?

Edited by

Tony Warne
Sue McAndrew

palgrave
macmillan

First published 2010 by
PALGRAVE MACMILLAN

Palgrave Macmillan in the UK is an imprint of Macmillan Publishers Limited, registered in England, company number 785998, of Houndmills, Basingstoke, Hampshire RG21 6XS.

Palgrave Macmillan in the US is a division of St Martin's Press LLC, 175 Fifth Avenue, New York, NY 10010.

Palgrave Macmillan is the global academic imprint of the above companies and has companies and representatives throughout the world.

Palgrave® and Macmillan® are registered trademarks in the United States, the United Kingdom, Europe and other countries.

ISBN-13: 978–0–230–57446–5

This book is printed on paper suitable for recycling and made from fully managed and sustained forest sources. Logging, pulping and manufacturing processes are expected to conform to the environmental regulations of the country of origin.

A catalogue record for this book is available from the British Library.

10 9 8 7 6 5 4 3 2 1
19 18 17 16 15 14 13 12 11 10

Printed in China

Contents

Acknowledgements

Peter Morrall would like to acknowledge the following colleagues for their help in moderating the more intemperate drafts of his chapter: Dr Jenny Wait-Jones and Jackie Ferguson, University of Leeds, UK, and Professor Mike Hazelton, University of Newcastle, Australia, for his continued critically supportive feedback regarding Peter's scholarly activities.

Cath Roper and Brenda Happell would like to acknowledge the involvement and support of Mr Ross Findlay and Ms Merinda Epstein, Melbourne Consumer Consultants' Group for their role in inspiring and developing the initial funding application. They also would like to thank Mr Bernie McCormack and Ms Margaret Yii, the consumer representatives, and Mr Greg Miller, the academic representative on the project team, for their contributions have made this work; the Commonwealth Department of Health and Aged Care, who provided the seed funding to make this position possible; finally the consumer participants in the Education and Training Partnerships in Mental Health, who changed their way of thinking forever. The authors and publisher would also like to thank D. Sesula for her permission to reproduce her poem 'You and Me', available at www.power2u.org.

Ann Gallagher and Andrew McKie would like to thank Professor Paul Wainwright, Dr Colin Macduff and the editors who read and commented upon earlier drafts of their chapter. The authors and publisher would also like to thank: Faber and Faber Ltd for permission to reproduce an extract from the poem 'As Expected' by Gunn, T. (1982) from *The Passages of Joy*, London: Faber and Faber; and both Saint Andrew Press and K. Stevens for permission to reproduce the poem 'Old Woman' by Stevens, K. (2000) from *Iona*, St Andrew Press.

Tony Warne and Sue McAndrew would like to thank the nursing students at the University of Leeds and Manchester Metropolitan University for allowing them to use their pictures as exemplars in their chapter.

Naomi Sharples would like to thank all the deaf qualified mental health nurses who have been the brave pioneers in this important undertaking. Also thanks must go those people in positions of power and influence who have supported the DPANE project by going beyond their current paradigm into new ways of thinking and being.

Mike Hazelton, Rachel Rossiter and Ellen Sinclair would like to thank the new graduate nurses and clinical nurse consultants who agreed to participate in this study. The study was at all times strongly supported by the Executive of the area mental health service involved in the study.

The project was in part supported by a grant from the Centre for Mental Health, NSW Health. Every effort has been made to trace the copyright-holders, but if any have been inadvertently overlooked the publishers will be pleased to make the necessary arrangements at the first opportunity.

Preface

This is a book aimed at those involved in preparing individuals to work in health and social care. In particular, the book is written for those who engage in the preparation of individuals for practice; for example, the university lecturer, the practice-based mentor, the vocational trainer or the advanced practitioner. The book is structured in such a way that it allows the reader to use it as a motivational resource in order to promote new ways of conceptualising and delivering education. Primarily the book focuses on raising awareness of the value of inter-subjectivity as a learning opportunity. Thus the book offers ways in which educators can better promote reflexivity through the use of self in the context of becoming a more effective educator, practitioner and person. Whilst this is an approach that can be found in many different professional contexts, it has most commonly been recognised as a fundamental aspect of mental health care. The contributors to this book are in the main practitioners, teachers, researchers and service users who have wide experience in mental health care. Indeed, the original drafts for the book were thus centred on mental health nursing. In reading these early drafts it became clear that the critical messages contained in these chapters have an appeal that would resonate with many others engaged in the provision of health and social care generally, whether as teachers, practitioners and/or recipients. The focus of the book was thus widened to reflect this emergent approach. Each chapter draws upon the 'real-life' experiences of the authors, as they have developed and refined more creative educational and practice development activities. Often these examples and case scenarios illustrate the different dimensions of learning and teaching by drawing upon experiences of students in training, qualified practitioners, service users and academics. All the chapters present lively debate that brings together a theoretical or conceptual perspective with the use of contemporary practice examples used in innovative education. Although many of the examples used retain their close connection with mental health care, the underlying principles easily translate into a variety of learning opportunities for those involved in health and social care.

Notes on Contributors

CHAPTER 1

Dr Peter Morrall has published provocatively on such subjects as madness, murder, sexuality and psychotherapy. He lives in (old) York, plays the saxophone and rides a motorbike (but generally not at the same time).

CHAPTER 2

Gary Rolfe is Professor of nursing at Swansea University. Gary researches and teaches philosophy, research methodology and reflexive practice to nurses and other health care practitioners and has published widely in these areas.

CHAPTER 3

Phil Barker is an artist, psychotherapist and Honorary Professor in the School of Medicine, Dentistry and Nursing, University of Dundee. He is Fellow of the Royal College of Nursing and was awarded *the Red Gate Award for Distinguished Professors* at the University of Tokyo in 2000. In 2008 he was voted one of the Top 20 Most Influential Nurses in the World in a UK public vote organised by *Nursing Times*.

Poppy Buchanan-Barker is Director of *Clan Unity International* – a consultancy focused on mental health recovery. She spent more than 25 years as a social worker with people with multiple disabilities and their families. She is also a counsellor in the areas of suicide, alcohol abuse and crisis resolution. In 2008 she was the joint winner of the *Thomas Szasz Award for Outstanding Contributions to the Cause of Civil Liberties* in New York.

CHAPTER 4

Timothy Wand is a nurse practitioner, mental health liaison, in the Emergency Department at the Royal Prince Alfred Hospital in Sydney, Australia, and Clinical Senior Lecturer in Mental Health at the Faculty of Nursing and Midwifery in the University of Sydney.

Brenda Happell is Professor of Contemporary Nursing at CQUniversity Australia. She is an active researcher with a strong publication record. She is currently the Editor-in-Chief of the *International Journal of Mental Health Nursing*, Associate Editor of *Issues in Mental Health Nursing* and a member of the Editorial Board for Mental Health and Substance Use and Psychosis.

Brenda is a member of the Board of Directors of the Australian College of Mental Health Nurses.

CHAPTER 5

Sam Samociuk trained as a psychiatric nurse in the 1970s, became interested in the further development of therapeutic approaches to mental health nursing, which involved him in personal development work and higher education, and became a full-time educator in the 1980s during the experiential learning revolution. A strong advocate for therapeutic interpersonal skills development and the need to embed clinical supervision as part of the concept of practice and as part of pre-registration education. Sam has championed service user and carer involvement in co-designing, planning and delivering joint perspectives in all aspects of educational provision in health and social care.

Anne Lawton has worked in the mental health field for over 20 years. She qualified as a nurse in the 1980s and went on to develop her interest in counselling and psychotherapy. She currently works as a mental health lecturer and as a counsellor in the voluntary sector. She is a strong advocate of developing counselling skills within nursing and is particularly interested in the interface between counselling and mental health nursing.

CHAPTER 6

Marie Crowe is Associate Professor holding a joint position with the Department of Psychological Medicine and the Centre for Postgraduate Nursing Studies, Christchurch, New Zealand. She is currently involved in a range of teaching and research projects and has a special interest in psychotherapy research and mood disorders.

CHAPTER 7

Cath Roper is Consumer Academic at the Centre for Psychiatric Nursing and Lecturer at the School of Nursing and Social Work, University of Melbourne. Cath is currently developing 'Proximity' – a consumer perspective academic programme with application to teaching and research activity.

CHAPTER 8

Ann Gallagher, at the time of writing, was Senior Research Fellow at Kingston University and St George's University of London. Ann is now Reader in Nursing Ethics and Director of the International Centre for Nursing Ethics at the University of Surrey. She recently completed the book *Ethics in Professional Life: Virtues for Health and Social Care* with Sarah Banks, University of Durham.

Andrew McKie is a lecturer in the School of Nursing and Midwifery at the Robert Gordon University in Aberdeen, Scotland. His teaching and research interests lie in the areas of mental health nursing, professional ethics and the use of the arts and humanities within professional health care education.

CHAPTER 9

Tony Warne is Head of School of Nursing, and Professor in Mental Health Care at the University of Salford, UK. He has over 30 years of experience in nursing practice, education and management. He has published extensively and is the Associate Editor of the *International Journal of Mental Health Nursing*.

Sue McAndrew has worked in mental health nursing for the past 30 years and is a trained marital and sex therapist. She has written extensively with Tony Warne, and co-edited 2 previous books. At the time of writing Sue was a lecturer at the University of Leeds, UK, but is now a research fellow at the University of Salford, UK.

CHAPTER 10

Gary Morris trained as a mental health nurse in the 1980s at Bexley hospital, Kent. His main clinical practice involved individual and group psychotherapy where he worked as an accredited Cognitive Analytic Therapist. He currently works as a mental health lecturer at the University of Leeds, where he teaches and runs modules across a wide professional spectrum but with a specific interest in Dementia care, Mental Health Issues and the Media, and Mentorship. In 2006 Gary published his first book, *Mental Health Issues and the Media*.

CHAPTER 11

Dr Margaret McAllister is Associate Professor in the School of Health and Sport Sciences at the University of the Sunshine Coast, Queensland, Australia. She is the programme leader for mental health studies. Her first book *Solution Focused Nursing: Rethinking Practice* was published in 2007 by Palgrave.

CHAPTER 12

Maureen Deacon has been involved in the development of mental health practice as a researcher, practitioner, educationalist, manager and leader. At the time of writing Maureen was the lead for continuing professional development in the Faculty of Health, Psychology and Social Care at Manchester Metropolitan University. Maureen is now a reader at the University of Chester.

CHAPTER 13

Professor Dawn Freshwater is Head of the School of Healthcare at the University of Leeds. Dawn has led research looking at practice innovations in prison health care and secure environments, suicide in young males and the psycho-social implications of Britain's ageing workforce. She is a fellow of the Royal College of Nursing and editor of the *Journal of Psychiatric and Mental Health Nursing*.

Dr Philip Esterhuizen is a lecturer at the Amsterdam School of Health Professions, Hogeschool van Amsterdam, the Netherlands. He is a reviewer for various nursing journals and has international experience in the areas of undergraduate and master's Curriculum Development. He has taught aspects of reflective practice and clinical supervision across settings and in different countries, and has been involved in developing clinical curricula based on reflective practice.

CHAPTER 14

Naomi Sharples is Director of Mental Health and Learning Disability Nursing at the University of Salford. She has worked with deaf people since 1993 and continues to explore new ways of developing inclusive education and employment practice for deaf people within the field of health and social care. Naomi's main area of teaching includes leadership, change management, reflective practice and diversity. Naomi's motivating heroes are Peter Senge, Paulo Freire and Archie, a coloured cob who provides equine therapy at just the right moments.

CHAPTER 15

Professor Mike Hazelton is Head of the School of Nursing and Midwifery and Professor of Mental Health Nursing at the University of Newcastle, Australia. He is a Life Member of the Australian College of Mental Health Nurses and has been heavily involved in teaching and researching mental health nursing for some 25 years.

Dr Rachel Rossiter is a clinician/academic with a broad range of clinical experience, including provision of mental health care at primary health care level, authorisation as a nurse practitioner in mental health and work experience as a psychotherapist. Rachel is currently employed as a project officer by the University of Newcastle, Australia, and continues active involvement in clinical work, providing clinical supervision to clinicians in a variety of clinical settings.

Ellen Sinclair is a former clinical nurse consultant in psychiatric rehabilitation in Hunter New England Mental Health Service, New South Wales, Australia. She is currently teaching mental health to undergraduate nursing students and completing a master's in Mental Health Nursing at the University of Newcastle, Australia.

Introduction

Tony Warne and Sue McAndrew

■ Challenging the traditions of 'taut' education

This book explores the value of finding new ways of teaching and learning the skills and knowledge required for contemporary health and social care. It was Georgi Lozanov (1979) who noted that learning was a matter of attitude and not aptitude. We argue that, equally, teaching and facilitating learning is also a matter of attitude and not just about aptitude. This book is aimed at stimulating thinking as to how students and practitioners might learn differently. This is not a book that simply suggests different ways to plan and facilitate a classroom lecture or clinical skills session, but is one that considers the philosophical approaches to health and social care education alongside the use of some engaging examples of approaches that can be considered in shaping the way professionals are prepared for future practice. As the traditional didactic transference of knowledge gives way to new approaches to teaching and changed expectations of students as to how their learning should be facilitated, it is often the attitude of individuals that determines the degree of resistance to or acceptance of such changes. In the context of acquiring and utilising knowledge for practice, learning from the theoretical and the emotional are interrelated, interactive and interdependent aspects of both individual functioning and professional practice. Together, these facets of learning are powerful sources of possible meaning and direction, supporting or inhibiting individual attempts to [re]define the reality of their everyday practice and their place within it (Antonacopoulou and Gabriel, 2001).

This book has its origins in what was a growing concern that, paradoxically, many traditional approaches to education have stifled creativity, innovation and the development of new world views. Being creative can be difficult and being a creative teacher can be just as difficult. Some of us would be located in a place where being creative is not a strength, albeit we might recognise the inherent creativity in a particular approach. Others might be located in a place where creativity is a normal aspect of their being, yet where such creativity is stifled by those who wish to be creative, but who are risk-adverse, and unconsciously seek stability and safety of the familiar. Interestingly, Chapter 11 explores how we might be able to learn from the familiar by taking a different look at what is often taken for granted. Of course, there will be others who don't want to be creative, because that is not what we were taught or shown to do.

The context for much of the work of contemporary university-based education is bounded by formulaic and ritualised approaches to teaching and learning. So, for example, the 'PhD student' is 'guided' through the intricacies of constructing a thesis that is in keeping with the cultural confines of academia yet is also often simultaneously expected to make a unique and innovative contribution to knowledge. Likewise, the ongoing theory–practice debate has borne testimony to how the health and social care students can struggle in trying to address the difference between what is taught as part of their academic course and what is experienced in practice. Such struggles often result in the student being discouraged from questioning their teachers and, as they move to gaining professional status, losing all motivation to resist the confining and debilitating habitus of professional practice (Scott, 2003). For some students the perpetuation of a theory–practice gap will only reassert what they perceive to be their already precarious position preventing them communicating and sharing their own ideas and beliefs, whilst others will passively adopt the attitudes of those they work with in practice. Such passivity reduces the opportunity for continuous and lifelong learning to influence and change practice.

Whilst we acknowledge that clinging to such formulaic familiar educational processes can provide security for some, often they do not provide a platform for exploring and synthesising the emotional knowing as integral to the development of the knowledge needed to deliver effective health and social care. Where the aim of contemporary health and social care education is to create reflective, analytical practitioners it is imperative that the appropriate teaching and learning processes and support systems are put in place in order that such individuals are able to flourish (Nolan et al., 1995). However, for some this remains little more than rhetoric (Freshwater and Stickley, 2004; Warne et al., 2007). It has been argued that the classroom is dominated by theoretical knowledge, with practical knowledge being the domain of clinical practice, and that education predicated on meeting statutory competencies is training rather than education (Freshwater and Stickley, 2004).

We argue that the contemporary preparation of health and social care practitioners requires a rethinking of the boundaries of traditional educational practice in order that we accommodate what might be contained in this emergent educational discourse. We have suggested elsewhere (Warne and McAndrew, 2007) that such rethinking requires conceptualising the dualistic nature of 'preparedness' as being both an educational and an emotional precept. In so doing, the possibility of addressing both the technical and theoretical knowledge required for practice and the attitudes and emotions that influence the individual *in* practice can be achieved.

This concept of preparedness also represents what we have described as the interrelated and entangling space between knowledge and knowing.

Just as theoretical knowledge is considered implicit in delivering good practice, knowing also forms part of our competence as it enables us to deal with our interpersonal relationships within the context of our external world. There is a discernible difference between 'knowledge' and 'knowing'. Knowledge has been described as a conscious secondary process relating to the information residing in one's mind, whilst knowing is the unconscious primary process, a product of our history which encompasses our beliefs and values, and is culturally and socially bounded (Reeder, 2002).

Thus it is our attitude to 'knowledge' and our aptitude for 'knowing' that allows us to explore and make sense of our own and other people's world in terms of experiences, feelings, needs and motives. The ability to 'know me' in order to better learn how to 'understand you' is the crux of the therapeutic relationship and is central to the notion of providing holistic care (see also End Note for a fuller exploration of these issues).

Chapter 5 explores the essential place developing therapeutic relationships has in health and social care practice (Crowe, 2004; Stickley and Freshwater, 2002). Such relationships require the individual care provider to be attentive, patient and attuned to hear the story and at the same time provide safety through containing both the story and the expressed personal *zeitgeist* of both the patient and the practitioner, thus making such relationships emotionally charged. It is through nurturance, caring about, love, compassion, respect, humanity, self awareness and mindfulness that the therapeutic effectiveness of these relationships is promoted (Stickley and Freshwater, 2002; McAllister, 2005; Barker and Buchanan-Barker, 2008). This book argues that in the student–teacher relationship such interpersonal dynamics are equally important if learning is to be creative and effective.

■ Knowing me and you

Experiential, interactive and inter-subjective learning activities provide opportunity for self-discovery and an increased understanding of personal meaning. Often when using such approaches, the emphasis is on identifying what contributes to or inhibits the effective use of self in relation to helping and/or working with others (Weissman et al., 2000). For many individuals such processes of self-examination and interpretation might be experienced as both threatening and confusing (Warne and McAndrew, 2007). This is perhaps understandable. We all favour knowing what it is we need to know in order to be the competent and effective health or social care professional we are expected to be. However, we want to suggest that perhaps it is that we yet *don't know* which might be important in terms of becoming and being an effective health and social care professional. For example, novice nurses, doctors and social workers complete their education and training possessing countless skills and much relevant theoretical knowledge. As educationalists we might be seen to have success-fully achieved our remit in preparing the future workforce for practice. Yet what many of these novice professionals lack is the knowing required to ensure such knowledge is used in a meaningful way with the uniqueness of the individuals they work with. It is as if the ability to work with others in a way that recognises the interpersonal dynamic of such relationships is missing.

Often in the educational process of becoming a nurse, a social worker, a physiotherapist and so on, the individual patient or client is relegated to the sidelines. Notions of self become lost in a mistaken desire to work 'skilfully' with others. One consequence of this is that we 'produce' individuals who are fit for the award they have studied for and fit for practice but, in terms of perhaps understanding the scope of what they should be doing, may not be fit for purpose. Chapter 3, for example, explores how often it can be diffi-cult to harness the knowledge gained in practice and the classroom in order to be able to make meaningful connections of the interpersonal encounters practitioners experience with those they are caring for. It is through devel-oping such meaning that values can then be conceived which synergistically augment one's sense of meaning (Yalom, 1980).

We suggest that creative teaching and learning approaches can pro-vide 'safe' ways of allowing students and practitioners to understand the relationship between using their theoretical and practice-based knowledge differently. This can be achieved by reflecting and recognising the impor-tance of another strand of knowledge. This is the patient experience knowledge and the emotionality of the interpersonal space these create between student and teacher, patient and practitioner. These three strands of knowledge are mediated by the individual's (practitioner) sense of self. A cohesive sense of self lays the foundation for discovering one's existence as a temporal being, capable of creating meaning. The greater this sense of a self is, the more likely it is that these strands of knowledge become knowing.

Winnicott's notion of a *holding* environment (Winnicott, 1971) and/or Bion's *containment* (Bion, 1963) both provide a conceptual approach to how the practitioner might free themselves from the limitations resulting from reliance, consciously or otherwise, on such ontological security. There is a parallel process here between what we expect of our students in clinical practice and what, as educationalists, we offer to our students in the edu-cational setting. Just as those in receipt of health and social care need to be nurtured, if we want to encourage our students to enter unfamiliar and uncomfortable places of being and learning, we will need to find ways of ensuring their humanity is nurtured.

Such nurturance will help facilitate the ability to develop a strong sense of self and not to be afraid of functioning as their true self. In achieving this status within the safe confines of the university, it is anticipated that when engaged in therapeutic practice they will be capable of productive meaningful work through their ability to share inner thoughts, feelings, beliefs, values and vision without fear of reprisal from the patient, colleagues and/or the organisation. It is a position marked by a moral courage that does not require educationalists to step back from society in the manner of the 'objective' teacher, but rather to distance themselves from those power relations that can often subjugate and oppress other human beings; in this instance, the student.

Asking the student to situate their self in relation to this experience provides an opportunity for students to safely deconstruct their experiences in terms of conceptual and experiential ways of knowing. Theoretical sense-making is dependent upon the knowledge, skill and experience of the tutor in being able to signpost, in a Socratian manner, those theories that might enable the student to anchor what for them might appear to be free-floating theories to the grounded reality of their practice experience and learning. Such a task could be seen as akin to Bion's notion of thoughts searching for a thinker, the unconscious encompassing transformations that may occur on the edges of chaos (the unknown), but which could be harnessed creatively through an effective learning encounter. However, the tutor's 'knowledge' and 'knowing' and attitude to 'not knowing' in this situation will impact not only on the effectiveness of the learning opportunity, but how the encounter is emotionally experienced by the tutor.

In moving towards new destinations, rather than remaining in that Plato's cave of familiarity and security but which provides only a limited view, we must turn, leave and face the unknown. In aspiring to achieve theoretical and emotional knowledgeable health and social care professionals, educators need to learn how to better listen to the students they work with in order to find out what it is they know and understand and use to make sense of the lives of the people they are working with and caring for. In so doing, educationalists will begin to learn what it is the student wants to achieve and what help is required in order to meet their learning needs. To expedite this would require a move away from a reliance on the delivery of pre-constructed theory as a way of promoting knowledge and understanding of the felt experience of patients and clients, towards a shared learning place, one where their patients, and the student, become the centre of their learning. Here, through creating opportunities for theory to be deconstructed, re-constructed and *fitted* accordingly, sense-making can be achieved (Warne et al., 2004). This is a notion congruent with the philosophical and pedagogical underpinnings to such approaches as lifelong learning.

In this introductory chapter we have started to develop the challenge for educationalists preparing people for working in the health and social arena to move away from the often formulaic and ritualistic familiar educational processes. Whilst we acknowledge that such processes provide security for all of those involved, they do not address the interrelated and entangled space between knowledge and knowing. We suggest that creative and innovative teaching and learning approaches can provide 'safe' ways of allowing health and social care students opportunities to explore the relationship between using their theoretical and practice-based knowledge in a way that both reflects and recognises the importance of the patient experience knowledge and the emotionality of the interpersonal space these create between patient and student. Where the aim of contemporary health and social care education is to create reflective, analytical practitioners it is imperative that the correct teaching and learning processes and support systems are put in place if we are to facilitate the development of professionals who are fit to practice.

References

Antonacopoulou, E. and Gabriel, Y. (2001) Emotion, learning and organizational change. *Journal of Organizational Change Management.* 14(5), 435–451.

Bion, W. R. (1963) *Elements of Psycho-Analysis.* London: Heinemann.

Barker, P. and Buchanan-Barker, P. (2008) Mental health in an age of celebrity: The courage to care. *Journal of Medical Ethics; Medical Humanities.* 34, 110–114.

Crowe, M. (2004) The place of the unconscious in mental health nursing. *International Journal of Mental Health Nursing.* 13, 2–8.

Freshwater, D. and Stickley, T. (2004) The heart of art: Emotional intelligence in nurse education. *Nursing Inquiry.* 11(2), 91–98.

Lozanov, G. (1979) *Suggestology and Outlines of Suggestopedy.* New York: Gordon and Breach, Science Publishers,

McAllister, M. (2005). Transformative teaching in nursing education: Preparing for the Possible. *Collegian.* 12(1), 13–18.

Nolan, M., Owen, G. and Nolan, J. (1995) Continuing professional education: Identifying characteristics of an effective system. *Journal of Advanced Nursing.* 22, 221–556.

Reeder, J. (2002) From knowledge to competence: Reflections on theoretical work. *International Journal of Psychoanalysis.* 83, 799–809.

Scott, G. (2003) Has nursing lost its heart? *Nursing Standard.* 18(13), 12–13.

Stickley, T. and Freshwater, D. (2002) The art of loving and the therapeutic relationship. *Nursing Inquiry.* 9(4), 250–256.

Warne, T., McAndrew, S., Hepworth, H., Collins, E. and McGregor, S. (2004) Looking back: Stepping forward. In: Warne, T. and McAndrew, S. (eds.) *Using Patient Experience in Nurse Education.* Hampshire: Palgrave MacMillan.

Warne, T., and McAndrew, S., King, M. and Holland, K. (2007) Rhetorical organisations of defense in primary care. *Primacy Health Care Research and Development.* 8(2) 183–192.

Warne, T. and McAndrew, S. (2007) Passive patient or engaged expert? Using a ptolemaic approach to enhance nurse education and practice. *International Journal of Mental Health Nursing.* 16, 224–229.

Weissman M., Markowitz, J. and Klerman, G. (2000) *Comprehensive Guide to Interpersonal Psychotherapy.* New York: Basic Books.

Winnicott, D. (1971) *Playing and Reality.* London: Routledge.

Yalom, I. D. (1980) *Existential Psychotherapy.* USA: Basic Books.

Part 1

Philosophy and Sociology of Health and Social Care Education

The first three chapters that make up this section are interrelated accounts that explore some familiar concepts and ideas in a way that hopefully challenges the reader to reflect upon the usefulness of such familiarity. Each of these challenges is presented differently. In Chapter 1, Peter Morrall provides an account that explores the explicit use of provocation in the educational process. Drawing on his wider experience as an educationalist and sociologist, he explores the changing nature of contemporary education and the almost unassailable move towards training as the preferred way of facilitating professional education. These themes are further developed by Gary Rolfe in Chapter 2. An incisive exploration of the way in which concepts of truth, validity and science have been misused by contemporary educationalists provides a challenging backcloth to a new way of thinking about how we should work with our students in preparing them for health and social care practice. The chapter explores the creation of knowledge and how this can be more effectively valued and contextualised, a theme further developed by Phil Barker and Poppy Buchanan-Barker in their Chapter 3. Here the use of narrative in the telling of an individual's story is explored. This chapter captures the essence of the concerns and issues set out in the first two chapters and provides a unique framework for many of the subsequent chapters as they seek to further explicate these issues.

Chapter 1

Provocation: Reviving thinking in universities

Peter Morrall

■ Introduction

There is a public health warning to this chapter: the content is deliberately controversial and challenging, and consequently it may upset some readers; however, the intention is not to be gratuitously offensive but to engage the reader and stimulate a response to the proposition set out here; what is proposed is that universities are no longer primarily about thinking but have become 'training warehouses' bogged down in bureaucracy, and that 'provocation' as a teaching tool can assist in the revitalisation of thinking; I invite the reader to deliver his/her response, whether supportive or antagonistic, to me personally (at p.a.morrall@leeds.ac.uk).

■ Provocation

Provocation in English Criminal Law can be used *defensively* in mitigation of murder of a human being. Here I campaign for the use of provocation *offensively* to reverse a murder – the killing of thinking in universities. Provocation-based learning has an extensive educational reach. Jon Mills (1998), for example, has argued that provocation can foster abstract thought, critical thinking, problem solving, and active/participatory learning. It can also, Mills suggests, be weaved into a Socratic 'cross examination' method through which conceptual inconsistency is exposed, thereby engendering clear thinking and intellectual progress. Mills was on a quest to encourage neophyte students to engage more effusively with his subject of philosophy.

Evolutionary psychologists and psychiatrists may postulate that provocation was socially functional to early human groupings. *Provocateurs*, the psycho-evolutionary theorists might muse, were catalysts for cultural progress, taking humanity further from the primordial pond and nearer to daytime television. Incitement challenged the presiding social order and norms of the tribe. Unless suppressed successfully (burning, boiling, or bashing being more popular than some latter-day control methods such as extensive incarceration), the consequence of provocation would be regular moderate modifications and occasional drastic alterations in how the tribe operated.

Provocation is core to the *modus operandi* of my chosen academic discipline and career, sociology. Since first starting to study sociology nearly 30 years ago, qualifying as a secondary/high school teacher in sociology, and then lecturing in sociology and health in higher education, it has been perpetually prodding and poking my thinking. In turn I've been prodding and poking the intellectual capacity of the students I teach and attempting to shape their intellectual capabilities.

Sociology has gained a reputation as an analytically critical discipline, and of analysing critically anything and everything. There are, for example, sociological specialists in religion, architecture, love, marriage, violence, sex, death, disease, and even McDonalds. Given my academic credentials I regard my primary function as an educator is to stimulate thinking.

But, despite my intellectual[1] and career commitments to sociology, I am not a sociological fundamentalist. It was the founding father of the discipline, August Comte (1798–1857), who declared that sociology was the 'last science'. As sociology would encompass all other fields of knowledge, Comte proposed that it therefore was the 'supreme' science (Comte, 1853). Sociology is essential, I suggest, to the understanding of both the natural and the social world (including the inner world of humans). But then so are many other disciplines. Moreover, as well as regular intellectual revelations, I accept there is considerable intellectual detritus discharged from sociology.

However, what I do regard fervently as an undeniable strength of the sociologist is an almost compulsive–obsessive impulse to ask challenging and discomforting questions about what are otherwise taken-for-granted ideas, values, and social edifices. Such provocations inevitably offend those with vested interests in what is otherwise accepted as true and moral (the power elites).

But my primary target for provocation here are not the power elites. By power-elites I am referring to those with centralised power (politicians, military dictators, and executives of global corporate and financial institutions), and localised power (the administrators of organisations, whether businesses, educational, criminal justice, or

---

[1] In case of doubt, I am not describing myself as an intellectual. However, I do indulge in thinking and respect those who think well.

health/social/medical care). The elites require different kinds of provocation such as that suggested by Marxist political theorist Antonio Gramsci (1891–1937). To undo the hegemony of the ruling class (that is the ideological infestation of the population by the ruling class with values that enhance the dominant position of that class) Gramsci (1971) expounded a 'war of position'. A 'war of position' implied a long and multifaceted campaign for the undoing of hegemony and thereby provoking political and cultural change. This Gramsci compared with the 'war of manoeuvre', a head-on assault against powerful people and their institutions. The concept of a 'war of manoeuvre' can also, I suggest, be used to describe what I term 'provocative pedagogy'. Indeed, Gramsci propounded a 'critical theory of education' to raise the political consciousness of students from the working class.

The vocational disciplines are particularly susceptible to political as well as intellectual atavism. But, students of all disciplines are psychologically dulled by the hegemony of global capitalism. That is, rather than conducting sit-ins in the Dean's and Vice Chancellor's office demanding some 'right' to be reinstated or 'cause' to be supported, they are more likely to be trapped by the rigours of contemporary assessment processes, and the materialism and employment requisites that effect everyone else. Students are no longer atypical of 'the system' but prototypical. What I am arguing for is the adoption of provocative pedagogy to raise intellectual consciousness, and political consciousness. What I mean by 'pedagogical provocation' is

A dramatic but defendable verbal, non-verbal, or written gesture intended to rouse or shift thinking significantly.

My quest is to provoke more attachment to *thinking* generally in universities but specifically amongst students and lecturers I have most contact with, those undertaking and teaching health/social/medical care courses (*and* their lecturers).

■ Aporia and truth

Attempting to understand the world, or even a selected element such as human health, is an intimidating and improbable educational mission even for the most intellectual lecturer and student. Additionally, the cerebrally disempowering exigencies of bureaucratisation, managerialism, instrumentalism, commodification, and consumerisation in our universities exacerbate the cognitively bewildering complexities created by the intricacies and vagaries of economic, scientific, environmental, social and political trends, quirks, advances, and catastrophes of global(ising) society.

Perhaps the best we can hope for is to be mindful of our ignorance *and* to be mindful that misunderstanding how ignorant we are can lead to personal and social tragedies. For example, misinformed and uninformed views about ethnicity, gender, age, or religion, the spread of infection, and the side effects of industrialisation are directly linkable to distress, disease, disorder, and death. We are now aware that water, fleas, and bad hygiene create epidemics, that fascism, racism, and tribalism can initiate genocide, and that the uncontrolled release of Co_2 is responsible for major climatic changes. With regard to what we know, what we don't know, and what we know we don't know *and* what we don't know we don't know, the precautionary principle should apply. But far from being cautious in our thinking in our universities, I suggest throwing caution to the wind, with provocation acting as the interlocutory gale that blows away intellectual temerity to reveal the state of our knowledge.

The Ancient Greeks, of course, have already prepared the intellectual ground concerning the shakiness of our knowledge. 'Aporia' in Greek philosophy is defined as having reached a state of perplexity and doubt regarding a seemingly established 'fact'. Socratic questioning is intended to lead either to the affirmation of a belief or to aporia. If the latter then the 'fact' may need to be rejected or more accurate understanding of the 'fact' may be worked towards.

Some considerable time after the heyday of Greek Philosophy came the postmodernists. The personification of postmodernism is the 'deconstructionism' of Jaques Derrida. Derrida (1993) borrowed the term 'aporia' from the Greeks and applied it to what he identifies are the confusions and paradoxes of our present-day lives. Derrida sought to expose the fallibility of seemingly factual phenomena (whether in the social or the natural world) and thereby 'deconstruct' virtually all accepted notions of reality. For him, ignorance, and the uncertainty that accompanies a realisation that we are ignorant, is the only reality. Furthermore, some questions (for example, about death) can never be answered rationally, and perhaps never should be attempted to be answered. Rather than searching for truth, argues Derrida, ignorance and uncertainty should be embraced and perhaps even enjoyed.

However, far from being intellectually enlightened, postmodernists such as Derrida have been derided for being '*intellectual impostures*' (Sokal and Bricmont, 1998). Whilst deconstructionist methods do have their usefulness in the examination of what is true and what is real, the deconstruction of all truth and reality (even war and death) leaves nothing but nihilism and inaction. For the sociologist Frank Furedi (2004), the search for truth remains a laudable if unachievable goal. Moreover, for Furedi, no matter how forlorn the search, truth is what universities should still be aiming to uncover. Without the search for truth universities have no *raison d'être* that makes them distinct from 'educational' establishments intended to train their attendees only in 'work skills' and provide them with 'applied knowledge'. Of course universities can and do offer students practical skills and knowledge, but without also wrestling with what is behind what is practical there is little point to the university.

Simon Blackburn (2006), Professor of Philosophy at Cambridge University, argues that truth and reality are worthwhile pursuits, but that we should be realistic about the likelihood of attaining this goal. Likewise, Brian Goodwin (2007), Professor of biology at the Open University, accepts that knowledge can only be an interpretation of reality because subjective opinions and social processes inevitably interfere with the search for facts. Goodwin wants the formation of a culturally sensitive and holistic science. But, the scepticism of these academics about truth is not equivalent to the cynicism of the postmodernists. The truth and reality of cancer, schizophrenia, loneliness, poverty, 'big-bang', the melting of the polar ice cap and destruction of the earth's ozone layer, and global financial crises can be examined for their cultural and political overtones and the robustness of the evidence to support their existence, but cannot be dismissed merely as social constructions (Morrall, 2009).

Admittedly, there is little 'evidence' to support the 'truth' that provocation can be a useful pedagogical tool. However, part of the stifling of thinking in universities arises from the narrowness of what counts as robust evidence. 'Empiricalitis' (the inflamed deification of experimental or observed data as the only indicators of truth: Morrall, 2009) has broken out in academic work (especially in the health and social domains). But empiricism is not the only way of looking at the world. Moreover, the crude variety of empiricism that has infested health and social care is virtually devoid of anything beyond superficial and tactical thinking. There is little opportunity to think deeply before deadlines have to be met for the submission of research proposals, the dissemination of research results, and the implementation of conclusions from research, particularly when it is politically expedient to do so.

Indeed, Furedi (2004) plaintively asks the question '*where have all the intellectuals gone?*' I am not arguing for the revitalisation of universities as '*ministries of mental masturbation*', what in effect they have traditionally been according to James Panton (2003) rather than hot beds for personal and social change. What I am suggesting is a critical teaching and political tool for combating both ignorance and apathy amongst students which provokes thinking, and thinking is a necessary precursor to action whether in relation to an individual's work and career or society overall. Panton suggests that provocation ('challenging' is his term) can have such wide function:

If those engaged in the pursuit of knowledge within the academy are prepared to challenge the current instrumentalist and philistine approach to higher education, they will also be challenging the conditions of intellectual apathy and disaffection in contemporary society more broadly.

This is a struggle that anyone who values the development of human knowledge and understanding cannot help but engage in. It is a struggle that is long overdue.

(Panton, 2003, p. 155)

■ Killing thinking

Intellectualism along with inspiration and initiative, I and others (for example, Panton) reason, are qualities of disrepute in today's universities, where the mavericks and activists have been weeded out through 'quality assurance', subdued by 'research exercises', constrained by 'work-load models', and forced to comply and compartmentalise by 'performance management'. What is left to furnish the former bastions of brain power and free-thinking is a business culture comprising of 'strategic planning' and an accompanying language which reinforces not the manufacture of ideas but the expansion of markets. Universities, like all other social institutions in Western society, have become hyper-regulated. The consequence of hyper-regulation in universities has been the insidious asphyxiation of the intellect. Within such constraints lecturers can often feel like assembly-line operatives in knowledge factories, cerebral endeavour being doped by the opium of mass education. Modules in mediocrity, with their blinkered and rigid learning and marking criteria, regurgitate pre-set propositions and paradigms in a self-sustaining teleological circle of pointlessness, thereby killing thinking for lecturer and student alike.

Thinking as an essential attribute in university education has all but disappeared. 'Provocation' is a direct, contagious, and dangerous, pedagogical approach to re-establish thinking as the foundation of all learning. Mary Evans (2004) writes fervently about the killing of thinking within British universities. Her argument is that intellectual vitality and creativity have been increasingly stultified since towards the end of the twentieth century:

.... since those years have seen the transformation of teaching in universities into the painting-by-numbers exercise of the hand-out culture and of much research into an atavistic battle for funds.

(Evans, 2004, p. ix)

University bureaucracy and managerialism is much worse than when Evans made her comments. The 'false-consciousness' of effectiveness and efficiency is more severe and steadfast, and hegemony more insidious and embedded. Genuine academic freedom has been curtailed under the oppressive and destructive forces of bureaucracy and managerialism. Genuine studentship has been buried under the duress of financial responsibility and indoctrinated with the ethic of work and accumulation.

Terry Eagleton (2008) is Professor of English Literature at Lancaster University and renowned social and literary critic. Eagleton was 'retired' by his previous employer, Manchester University, where he states that he had been originally employed to perform '*as a kind of maverick*' but subsequently, according to Eagleton, the university authorities '*didn't seem able to cope with it*' (Eagleton in Gill, 2008). Moreover, his '*retirement*' coincided with major financial readjustments at Manchester University which threatened hundreds of jobs. Eagleton suggests that universities have ceased to enact their classical role as the principal agencies of social critique as well as knowledge production, and have become part of the capitalist mode of production. By and large, universities have shifted from being accusers of corporate capitalism to being its accomplices. They are, for Eagleton, 'intellectual Tescos' churning out a commodity known as graduates rather than greengroceries (Eagleton, 2008, p. 16).

Naturally, such a position is contestable. It can be argued that such critics (including myself) of the present university *modus operandi* are merely malcontents who would complain about any organisational or 'reactionaries' fearful of change, and that all academics have to 'live in the real world'. Furthermore, the contra-position may continue, understanding the 'real world' has to be 'evidence-based' (using empirical data). Those in the health and social care disciplines may argue that for them the move into universities is an indication of occupational advancement, and that what they now receive is both training *and* education (including time and opportunity to think). However, neither the existence of malcontents nor the assumed benefits from being subsumed within the university system remove the potency of the central point that the overall effect of the trends identified by Eagleton, Evans, Furedi, and Panton is that the furthering of thinking is no longer the core justification for the existence of universities. Furthermore, 'the real world' is precisely what academics should be *thinking* about and then (and only then) advocating amendments to that world based on perhaps empirical evidence but also on other forms of knowledge, such as the result of reasoned debate.

What Eagleton advocates is the emergence of a new generation of intellectuals who can contribute effectively to society. What I'm urging of both established and neophyte academics is the re-adoption of dynamic critical commentaries in their writing, lectures, seminars, and conferences, as well as engaging in political debate and action.

■ Provocative types

As with any revolutionary paradigm shift (and reviving thinking back in universities is a revolutionary paradigm shift even if there is a return to key principals of former times), there have to be self-selecting *agent provocateurs* whose mission is to fuel discord in order to inspire change. My favourite provocateurs are those who posit sensational social commentary. Political economist Karl Marx continues to terrify the governing classes with his exposition on the exploitative nature of capitalist economic production. Philosophical historian Michel Foucault's iconoclastic proclamation that 'all knowledge is ridden with power' has done much to undermine the authority of those groups (for example, medicine, the law) that promote their 'discourse' as 'reality'.

Liberation theologian and Priest Gustavo Gutiérrez Merino has campaigned against corruption, injustice, and poverty in South America much to the chagrin of the Catholic Papacy. Paulo Freire was an innovative educator who advocated an 'informal teacher–student cooperation' to 'build a pedagogy of the oppressed'. A consequence of this pedagogical cooperation would be the emergence of what Gramsci (1971) termed 'organic intellectuals' (distinguishable from the traditional and elitist intellectuals) to lead society towards equitability, and that disturbed the Italian fascist regime of Benito Mussolini so much that he was given a very long custodial sentence.

However, sociologist, political philosopher, script writer, and charismatic ranter Slavoj Žižek is for me the ideal typification of a *pedagogical provocateur*. Like others mentioned above, Žižek has also managed to upset quite a lot of people including feminists, postmodernists, and liberals at various points in his intellectual and media career. More recently, Žižek's apparent support of the terror tactics of Robespierre and Lenin and for '*liberated territories*' has rattled fellow Marxists. Indeed Žižek's provocation knows no bounds, including the indictment of anyone with a philanthropic leaning. Žižek combines humour and substantive knowledge within his writing and presentations. His biographer Tony Myers observes of Zizek:

> [H]e thinks and writes in such a recklessly entertaining fashion.... With a happy disregard for the typically cloistered atmosphere of critical thought, Zizek's is frentic and explosive.
>
> (Myers, 2003, p. 1)

Moreover, Zizek uses 'constant amazement' as both a verbal and a non-verbal challenge to his audiences. He wants the audience to think 'why are things like that?' Zizek wants to examine everything not just straight on but sideways, above, below, and behind. There needs to be more Zizeks in the classroom.

■ Principles and precautions

The aim of pedagogical provocation is, therefore, to revive thinking by applying a psychological defibrillator to the dead intellectual heart of the health and social care disciplines who find themselves constrained by the modern university. The result may not be a full-blown paradigm replace-ment, but at the very least students will be more intellectually alive than they had been.

For educationalists to be triumphant in provocative pedagogy certain per-sonal qualities and skills are required. Many, if not most, of these proposed provocative attributes defy what has become the accepted discourse relating to teaching and learning (which, of course, is the point):

1. *Ostentatious exuberance*: The provocateur has to be self-assured and tena-cious at first with his/her arguments but then when responded he/she has to shift to a style reminiscent of Socratic questioning – constantly asking the question 'why'.
2. *Comedic incisiveness*: Humour, irony, and satire are indispensable aca-demic virtues when juxtaposed with provocative propositions.
3. *Fearless erudition*: Expert knowledge is paramount; the *provocateur* has to know his/her subject extremely well, and be prepared to go boldly where no one else has gone by extending the possibilities of both his/her knowledge and the potential of his/her audience.

A commitment to raising the intellectual consciousness of others through provocation demands a mixture of assuredness in one's own thinking capacity, skilled application of the technique, and bravery. With regard to the latter, the law of unexpected consequences applies. Volatile and hostile reactions may occur. However, the shape and scale of reactions cannot be predicted, and it is necessary that this is so. Otherwise, all the supposed *provocateur* is accomplishing is further management and bureaucratisation of the learning process and this is the very aspect of university education that he/she is trying to reveal an escape route from.

Although attempting to provide 'outcomes', a requirement for all present-day university teaching input, is an anathema to the aim of ped-agogical provocation, alterations in levels of participation in the class-room can be measured as can the quality of assessed work. Increased involvement by students, whether in the form of objections, questions, or statements in lectures or discussions during seminars and tutorials, and more in-depth critical analysis and synthesis in essays and examinations following provocation can be intentional and tangible outcomes of the strategy. These must not be achieved at the expense of unintentional and intangible outcomes that provocation is designed to incite. As you will see in other chapters of this book, paradoxically, processes that ideally should not contain quantifiable outcomes can enhance module and course objectives.

Patently, not every educationalist is cut out to be a provocateur and provocation needs to be targeted well. The provocateur has no detailed manual to use as a guide or specialised course to attend through which a qualification in provocation could be awarded. Such a guide or course would be counter-productive because inevitably it would be prescriptive. Trial and error is the mainstay of practising provocation. Practical class-room tips, such as they are, include starting at a relatively low level of provocation and with experience building up to more substantial exper-imentation. Selecting certain sessions and subjects is likely to be more effective than bombarding students with provocations at every opportu-nity. Self-reflection regarding how well a session with the students went is necessary, and appropriate adjustments can then be made. A danger for the academic utilising provocation is, because it is emotionally and intellectually demanding and idiosyncratic, he/she may feel isolated and vulnerable. The support of colleagues both within one's own institution and the wider academic community is important as is the sharing of ideas about technique and regarding any 'fall-out' from classroom interactions or managerial interventions.

It is recommended that those responsible directly for the running of the relevant student programmes are informed to ensure that even if they do not agree with the method they are aware of its pedagogical rationale and also can exercise their right to veto its use. Their veto may be employed on the grounds that they do not accept the pedagogical legitimacy of provoca-tion, or they regard the 'danger' to students as too great, such as individual students becoming too angry or confused about what is happening in the classroom when provocation is taking place.

■ Provocative example from practice

I have chosen the following example of my academic provocation because it covers both classroom activities and work I have published, and a wide range of students come into contact with this particular provocative input (as well as other fellow academics where I have been invited to present this material).

☐ The trouble with therapy

That therapists belong to an undisciplined, immature, and immoral enter-prise is the challenge I tender to students undertaking various therapy modules or courses as well as to the therapy enterprise as whole in my book titled *The Trouble With Therapy* (Morrall, 2008). In the classroom and in the book the following is proposed:

> The therapy enterprise has a long history of conflicts and rivalries which remain today, and choosing a type of therapy and a therapist is a lottery. Therefore, therapy is a deeply dysfunctional discipline.

The therapeutic enterprise has become arrogant about efficacy. Therapy is being steadily legitimised through the application of science. That is, there has been a 'scientisation' of therapy. But science is a conceited discourse (and, by association, so is therapy). Apart from serious flaws in the politics and procedures of science, the scientific fallacy is that reality can be explained.

Therapy is 'selfish' because it has overwhelming focus on the 'self' and omits to examine the external influences on human performance. The self is not only in a 'reflexive' relationship with society but is becoming saturated and sexualised by society.

Therapy is abusive because whilst empowerment is claimed to be at the heart of therapy, the therapeutic enterprise – institutionally, intellectually, and interpersonally – has a disempowering effect on its clientele. Moreover, therapy is an agency of social control.

Therapy is becoming '*infectious*' in a similar way to how '*medicalisation*' has become disabling. '*Therapyitis*' undermines the individual's ability to take care of his/her own problems of living, and makes society dependent on therapists to sort out social problems.

The business of therapy is madness, but it has limited knowledge of the medical history and discourse of madness, having virtually no knowledge of how society impinges on sanity. This in itself is a form of madness.

Therapy claims happiness is possible, and wants clients to be happy (or at least less miserable). But, that therapy can allay globalised inequality, disease, pollution, and violence is a grand and immoral deceit.

These 'seven sins of therapy' are exposed to students at undergraduate and post-graduate levels. Some of the students are undertaking courses in mental health nursing or social work, whilst others are participants in specialist therapy programmes (and who may already be experienced therapists). Once the students are emotionally and intellectually 'warmed up' and grappling with what they frequently consider prejudicial and unjustified criticisms (although some will agree that the sins have legitimacy), I then aim to introduce the more sophisticated reasoning that lies behind these seemingly vicious attacks on therapy and point out that rather than statements they are questions ('Is therapy dysfunction?', etc.). On occasions, the initial stage has produced highly heated exchanges between myself and the students and/or between students, and the second stage has either been delayed or, very rarely, not reached at all (another danger countered to some degree by suggesting further reading and/or further opportunities for debate). During both stages, as the educator my task is not only to talk but to listen, and in doing so provide at an opportune moment a summary of what has been presented and of the responses (this can be achieved verbally or electronically). Ideally this can lead to a 'synthesis' of ideas, thereby providing teacher and student with new understandings.

■ Conclusion

For Panton (2003), '*training*' rather than education is the trend in contemporary universities because vocationalism has become blurred with higher learning (much of which concerns the ability to think). Moreover, certain vocational university programmes are particularly susceptible to the repression of cognition. The hyper-regulation of health and social care courses can often stifle thinking. Nurses, social workers, audiologists, medical practitioners, and therapists have (or rather are supposed) to abide by the rules of the academe but also the rules of their respective occupational training bodies, and are trained in the overt and covert rules of the practice areas they partake in as part of their course. So, notwithstanding the inclusion of '*thinking*' in one guise or another within the philosophy and content of some of these courses, both the educator (trainer) and the educated (trained) are hide-bound by an embarrassment of conventions that mitigate thinking. Provocation, however, can be utilised as an educational tool to help combat the chains of hyper-regulation and thereby allow the freeing of thinking or at least for free-thought to be given a day-pass to visit what Zizek (2008) describes as 'liberated territories', havens of living thinking into which thinkers can migrate and from which thoughts can proliferate.

References

Comte, A. (1853) *The Positive Philosophy* (translated by Martineau, M). London: Trubner.

Derrida, J. (1993) *Aporias* (translated by Dutoit, T). Stanford, USA: Stanford University Press.

Eagleton, T. (2008) Death of the Intellectual. *Red Pepper*, 162 October/November, pp. 16–17.

Evans, M. (2004) *Killing Thinking: The Death of the Universities*. London: Continuum.

Furedi, F. (2004) *Where Have All the Intellectuals Gone?: Confronting 21st Century Philistinism*. London: Continuum.

Gill, J. (2008) *Eagle Lands: Literary Critic Snapped Up by Rivals After Forced Retirement*. Times Higher Education, 23rd October. http://www.timeshighereducation.co.uk/story.asp?sectioncode=26&storycode=404014.

Gramsci, A. (1971) *Selections from the Prison Notebooks*. Translated & Edited: Hoare, Q. & Smith, G. N. New York: International Publishers.

Mills, J. (1998) Better Teaching through Provocation. *College Teaching*, 46 (1), 21–25.

Morrall, P. (2008) *The Trouble With Therapy: Sociology and Psychotherapy*. Bucks: Open University.

Morrall, P. (2009) *Sociology and Health*. London: Routledge.

Myers, T. (2003) *Slavoj Žižek*. London: Routledge.

Panton, J. (2003) What Are Universities For? Universities, Knowledge and Intellectuals. *Critical Reiew of International Social and Political Philosophy*, 6 (4), 139–156.

Zizek, S. (2008) *Violence*. London: Profile.

Chapter 2

Back to the future: Challenging hard science approaches to care

Gary Rolfe

■ Introduction

This chapter explores the challenges involved in developing creative approaches to health and social care education and practice through an examination of the ways that the health and social care disciplines chose to position themselves when they entered higher education during the second half of the previous century. In particular, I will argue that many of the health and social care disciplines aligned themselves with the practical emancipatory project of science just at the time when academic science was moving away from pragmatic concerns about freeing individuals from pain and suffering towards a more transcendent quest for Truth (with a capital T).

As we shall see, this shift in focus from the specific 'little narratives' of human suffering towards establishing the scientific method as the overarching 'metanarrative' (that is, as the only valid route to the Truth) has resulted in some serious impediments to creative knowledge production and dissemination. Firstly, the metanarrative of science has enforced the rigorous adherence to certain research methodologies as the only way of producing 'valid' findings. This, we might argue, has stifled and discredited some of the more creative approaches to generating knowledge in the health and social care disciplines. Secondly, science has imposed a particular one-way 'denotative' approach to communicating these research findings which requires of the receiver only that they listen and act on what they have been told. And thirdly, science has lately striven to suppress the truth claims of the arts and humanities as of no consequence (or even as a danger) to the concerns of the health and social care disciplines. In short, recent changes in the focus and goals of science are in danger of leaving health and social care education as merely a one-way conduit between authoritative and sometimes authoritarian researchers and passive and complicit technicians.

Creative approaches in health and social care education can be effectively introduced only if educationalists have mutual, bilateral relationships with the knowledge producers (researchers and theorists) on the one hand and the knowledge appliers (students and practitioners) on the other. Whereas most chapters in this book focus on the latter relationship, this chapter examines the former. Furthermore, it points out that, in higher education, the educationalists are usually also the researchers, and urges us all to rethink our attitudes and relationships to the generation, communication and application of knowledge for effective practice.

■ Education and the Enlightenment project

Health and social care education (as distinct from training or apprenticeships) is a relatively new development in the UK, and came of age with the move into the higher education sector during the 1980s and 1990s. This move towards all-graduate professions was, of course, partly driven by political expediency (and was accompanied by a largely right-wing political backlash),[1] but also had a significant symbolic component. Thus, albeit two centuries late, the health and social care disciplines finally signed up to the Enlightenment project and, by definition, joined the modern age.

In order to understand the full significance of this modernisation or 'coming of age' of health and social care, we need to consider the key role played by the University (as an institution) following the scientific revolution of the seventeenth century and the subsequent 'age of Enlightenment' in the arts and sciences. For Readings (1996), the primary role of the modern University[2] has been as the generator and carrier of culture; indeed, culture has been 'the animating principle of the University'. Lyotard (1984) suggests that the modern University has traditionally told two different stories in order to justify or validate its role in the generation and dissemination of knowledge and culture. These 'grand narratives of legitimation' are the speculative, which promotes knowledge as an end in itself with universal truth (that is, Truth with a capital T) as its goal, and the

---

[1] For example, when nursing entered higher education in the UK in the 1990s, Brian Sewell complained about the 'appalling waste' of degree level education when applied to the work of nurses at 'bedpan level', a view echoed by the Conservative politician Anne Widdecombe, who was concerned about who was now going to empty the bedpans. In a similar vein, Nigel Lawson denounced the move of nursing into higher education as a 'ludicrous proposition', whilst Melanie Phillips complained that nursing was being contaminated by 'the nihilistic, politically correct gibberish that has disfigured social sciences' (all cited in Payne, 1999).

[2] Readings traces the birth of the modern University (with a capital U) to Humboldt's early-nineteenth-century prototype of the University of Berlin.

emancipatory, which argues that knowledge is merely a means to the end of universal freedom and justice.

Until relatively recently, the former of these grand narratives of legitimation has been largely regarded as the province of the arts and humanities faculties of the University. The arts in particular have for many centuries been charged with the exploration and expression of Truth, a view exemplified in Keats' declaration that 'Beauty is truth, truth beauty.' Similarly, William Blake believed that the 'eternal realities' were not to be discovered in the outside world through empirical science, but exist in the human imagination. Thus

> If it were not for the Poetic or Prophetic Character, the Philosophic [i.e. scientific] and Experimental would stay still unable to do other than repeat the same dull round over again.
>
> (Blake, 1788/1927, p. 64)

More recently, Picasso has expressed the view that 'art is a lie that helps us see the truth'. It is a lie insofar as it does not offer us a faithful correspondence with the realities of the external world, and yet it somehow provides us with access to a larger Truth about the human condition.

In contrast, the sciences have, until recent times, been concerned with the second of Lyotard's grand narratives of legitimation. For Lyotard, this emancipatory narrative has its origins in the French Revolution and with the ideals of universal education and the power of science to reduce suffering and transform society. This narrative promotes knowledge as a means of improving quality of life, and has traditionally been encountered most often in University faculties of the natural, biological, social and political sciences. So, for example, the industrial revolution, one of the earliest and most significant products of applied science, is noted *not* for its contribution to truth, but for the emancipation of the 'common man' (the emancipation of the 'common woman' followed much later) from the drudgery and hand-to-mouth existence of pre-industrial agricultural life. A similar position was taken by Karl Marx, who believed that science could, if used wisely, free the oppressed workers from the shackles of their labours, although he cautioned that it could also be misappropriated by the capitalist ruling classes as a means of further oppression and control. Likewise, the immense contribution made by science to medicine over the past two centuries was driven less by a desire for truth than to emancipate humankind from pain and premature death. It could, of course, be argued that the two aims are inseparable, that medical progress depends on uncovering the Truth, but, as I shall argue later, this presupposes a very narrow and empiricist 'correspondence theory of truth'.

We should be careful not to be too rigid in our distinction between the traditional narratives of legitimation for the arts and sciences. The humanities in particular have made valid claims for utility and the sciences and even Galileo recognised the limitations of the scientific method as a road to Truth:

> I know very well that one single experiment or conclusive proof to the contrary would be enough to batter to the ground a great many probable arguments.
>
> (Galileo, 1629/1967, p. 74)

Galileo was clearly aware that science was not dealing in universal and eternal Truths, but merely in provisional knowledge. In fact, he is expressing above the so-called 'problem of induction', which suggests that the inductive method of science (the accumulation of observations or cases) can *never* result in certainty and truth, since it is always open to later revision. Or, to put it in Galileo's terms, it takes an infinite number of positive observations to prove a theory by induction, but only one negative observation to disprove it.

Thus, when Auguste Comte attempted in the Nineteenth Century to apply the model of the physical sciences to human social behaviour, he recognised that the recent spectacular successes of physics and chemistry were due to the focus of these sciences on technological advance rather than on the quest for universal Truth. His 'positive science' (what came to be known as positivism) therefore 'gives up the search after hidden causes of the universe and a knowledge of the final causes of phenomena' (Comte, 1830/1988), arguing that the search for these 'underlying causes' (or what we might term 'fundamental truths') is 'absolutely inaccessible and unmeaning'.

The economist Milton Friedman summarised Comte's positivism as 'the development of a "theory" or "hypothesis" that yields valid and meaningful (i.e. not truistic) predictions about phenomena not yet observed' (Friedman, 1968). Positivism, as originally formulated, was therefore concerned with *useful predictions* about how the world works rather than statements of what is *true*. Pratt (1978) goes even further to suggest not only that 'the truth of a theory's assumptions should not enter into the assessment of its values', but that 'truth in assumptions actually *gets in the way* of predictive capacity'. Thus, for the positivists, where there is a conflict between the 'truth' of a theory and its usefulness, we should opt for utility.

More recently, the twentieth-century philosopher of science Karl Popper has postulated a post-positivist 'hypothetico-deductive' method of scientific enquiry, in which hypotheses are tested in order to disprove them. Theories therefore compete in what he likens to a process of Darwinian evolution, in which the last theory left standing (the 'fittest' theory) is the one that we should adopt. His point, however, is that any theory is open to being disproved at any time, and thus the notion of inviolable scientific laws and absolute scientific Truths is a myth. Thus 'we must regard all laws or theories as hypothetical or conjectural; that is, as guesses' (Popper, 1972). This, as he continued, is not to say that some of our theories might not be true; it is just that we can never be sure.

It is perhaps becoming clear, then, that the scientific method, in both its inductivist and its hypothetico-deductivist forms, was designed to produce *useful* and *workable* hypotheses and theories, and its only legitimate claims to Truth have been in the pragmatic sense that 'the truth is what works best' (James, 1907/1995). Thus, the main purpose of science has traditionally been to make the world a better place, with the exploration of Truth being generally left to the artists. However, it could be argued that, increasingly, science is failing to keep to its side of the bargain; that it is encroaching into a territory that has traditionally been the province of the arts.

■ The new dark ages

Even a cursory glance at the history of the Western world since the beginning of the Enlightenment will reveal that the scientific project of promoting efficiency and effectiveness has the potential for misuse. For Lyotard, the misappropriation of science from a tool of emancipation to one of suppression reached its nadir with the systematic and technological murder of millions by the Nazis during the Second World War. As Readings (1991) puts it, 'the summit of reason, order, administration, is also the summit of terror'. Thus, for Lyotard, 'Auschwitz can be taken as a paradigmatic name for the tragic "incompletion" of modernity' (Lyotard, 1992). Arguably, then, the post-war years have witnessed an abandonment (or at least a revision) of the Enlightenment values and the dawn of what MacIntyre (1985) has termed the 'new dark ages'. Over the past 50 years, science has been rebranded as a 'pure' discipline and scientists as remote and disinterested objective seekers after truth. Many scientists would claim that they simply provide value-free knowledge and it is politicians or society as a whole which then decides whether that knowledge will be used for good or evil. This attitude allowed Einstein to disclaim all responsibility for the invention of the hydrogen bomb, claiming that had he known the use to which his work would be put, he would have become a watchmaker. Arguably, then, the legitimating narrative of science, its *raison d'être*, has shifted from the pragmatic concern over effectiveness and emancipation to the pure and unsullied quest for Truth.

■ Science as a metanarrative

Lyotard (1984) suggests not only that the modern University has employed narratives or stories in order to legitimate its quest for knowledge, but that knowledge itself is organised and disseminated through a variety of different types of narrative. These are the 'language games' (Wittgenstein,

1958) that we use to tell stories about what we know, and include the denotative (describing), the performative (acting out through language), the prescriptive (giving orders), the interrogative (asking questions) and so on.

Lyotard suggests that modern science has come to rely on a single form of narrative underpinned by the language game of denotation or description. Furthermore, in its scientific guise, this form of narrative is different from most others in a number of ways. Most importantly, the scientific denotative narrative has become divorced from its social origins in oral storytelling. Thus, unlike other forms, scientific narratives do not have to be heard and accepted by their audience in order to gain validity: 'within the bounds of the game of research, the competence required concerns the post of sender [of the narrative] alone' (Lyotard, 1984). Scientific knowledge, unlike other forms, is validated solely through the status of the researcher and by adherence to the scientific method. Science has therefore become a 'metanarrative', a *self-validating* story which does not require a listener or a reader to validate its truth-claims, but which is true, simply by demonstrating its rigorous adherence to its own self-appointed rules.

This scientific view of the generation and communication of knowledge has some profound and far-reaching implications for health and social care education. The denotative metanarrative employed by modern science suggests that education is a one-way process of communication from master to pupil, and that the receiver of the message has no role to play in accepting and validating the message: it is for the scientist to demonstrate, usually through adherence to an accepted methodology, that the work is valid and truthful. In contrast, the narratives employed in education in the arts and humanities such as the interrogative and the performative require an active response from the student (and more generally from society) in order to firstly accept the message, and secondly to validate it, an idea further explored in Chapters 7 and 8. Education within the metanarrative of science, however, requires the student to merely accept, memorise and apply the message to practice.

However, the problem runs deeper than simply the choice of narrative form employed by the metanarrative of science to communicate and educate. More and more often during the past century, scientists have been making claims not only for uncovering the Truth, but that the metanarrative of science is the *best* or even the *only* method for uncovering the Truth. This latter view, characterised as 'Elevating scientific truth to Truth with a capital T' (Ridley, 2001), has been referred to as 'scientism', which has perhaps reached its apotheosis in the writing of Richard Dawkins, for whom 'Science is the only way we know to understand the real world' (cited in Midgely, 2001). On the face of it, this claim is nonsense since there are numerous ways of understanding the 'real world' apart from the scientific, including the methods and practices of the arts and humanities. In fact, the only way that Dawkins' claim can stand up to scrutiny is if the very definition of what is 'real' and what is meant by 'understanding' is narrowed down to just that which is revealed by empirical observation. This view is known as the correspondence theory of truth, where a statement can be said to be true if and only if it corresponds to our observations of the outside world. The scientist Richard Feynman clearly expresses this view when he claims that science is 'based on the principle that what happens in nature is true, and is the judge of the validity of any theory about it' (Feynman, 1999). From here, it is a short step to argue that science provides us with the most (or even the only) methodical and objective way of observing the outside world, and thus the scientific method offers unique access to the Truth.

Clearly, such a circular argument provides the method of science with a *de facto* monopoly on truth-claims. From the scientific perspective, art is not only a lie, but it has no relationship whatsoever with the Truth. This allows the scientist to make a clear and unilateral distinction between the metanarrative of science and all other 'little narratives'. Thus the scientist

> classifies [little narratives] as belonging to a different mentality: savage, primitive, underdeveloped, backward, alienated, composed of opinions, customs, authority, prejudice, ignorance, ideology. Narratives [other than science] are fables, myths, legends, fit only for women and children.
>
> (Lyotard, 1984, p. 27)

We can perhaps discern this sentiment in a number of criticisms levelled by the scientific community at those practitioners and academics who resist the 'hard science' approach of the evidence-based practice movement, as, for example, when Phillips (1994) describes all midwifery practice not based on empirical research as being based on 'folklore'.

This line of reasoning has been employed to condemn entire disciplines of health and social care practice, which are perhaps not amenable to being tested by randomised controlled trials. However, even in those disciplines such as nursing, which has attempted to engage with the evidence-based movement, the rejection of any knowledge not deriving from scientific research as 'fable, myth and legend' severely limits the scope for creative education based on the arts and humanities. There is no room for the novel or the poem as a *bona fide* source of knowledge, no opportunity to explore the truth of painting in relation to health care, and a playing down of the personal and experiential knowledge and insights gained from reflection and role-play.

I have suggested, then, that science has lost its way, that it has become derailed from pursuing its original emancipatory aim. In so doing, it has distorted and narrowed the very concept of truth to (self-referentially) what can be proved by science. This change in the aims and purpose of science has been comparatively recent, and yet it is already difficult to think of science as anything other than the principal methodology in the quest for Truth, whilst the role of the arts appears to have been relegated in status to little more than entertainment. Empirics has taken over from aesthetics as the royal road to Truth, and this shift has had profound implications for health and social care practice and hence for the ways in which practice is taught in the University. In particular, the emphasis on scientific knowledge to the exclusion of all else has served to stifle creative approaches to health and social care education.

■ Health and social care practice in the academy

We have seen that the modern University traditionally made the distinction between aesthetic knowledge, which underpinned the grand narrative of truth, and empirical scientific knowledge, which drove the grand narrative of emancipation. Clearly, the health and social care professions require both. In some cases, practitioners need to understand the existential or lived truth of the experiences of their clients, and it is here that the Arts and Humanities have generally been of greatest help. For example, whereas empirical research provides us with important information about populations, the study and use of novels, poetry and plays as can be seen in the issues discussed in Chapters 3, 7 and 9, can offer greater insights into individual situations and characters which often resonate with our own experiences (Rolfe, 2002). As the linguist and social scientist Noam Chomsky observed,

> It is quite possible – overwhelmingly probable, one might guess – that we will always learn more about human life and human personality from novels than from scientific psychology.
>
> (Chomsky, 1988, p. 159)

As Brown (1994) put it, both the textbook *Celestial Navigation* and the novel *Moby Dick* might contain useful knowledge for a sea voyage, 'respecting the validity of each for their specific purposes'.

But clearly, whatever the origins of health and social care knowledge, it is almost always regarded as a means to the end of helping the client to improve their life in some way. Thus, when the health and social care disciplines negotiated their entry into the University, most chose to make their homes in the faculty of science. This, I would argue, is absolutely right since the overtly stated aim and philosophy of most of the health and social care disciplines is *not* primarily the pursuit of Truth but the practical emancipation from suffering in one form or another.

However, I believe that in many cases health and social care academics have made two fundamental errors in the way they have positioned themselves in the University. On the one hand, they have adopted an inappropriately 'hard' scientific paradigm that does not address the needs of health and social care practitioners in improving their practice. On the other hand, some health and social care academics have become seduced by the (false) promise that the methods of the 'hard sciences' can lead beyond utility and emancipation to the discovery of Truth. Indeed, a few have fully embraced the philosophy of scientism and claim that the hard sciences provide the *only* path to truth. As we have seen, each of these errors has profound implications for the educational process in health and social care.

■ Utility, truth and pragmatism

I have suggested that the relatively short history of health and social care research has witnessed a growing focus on the scientific quest for universal Truth through the rigorous application of method. One of the first academics to express concern about this was the educationalist Lawrence Stenhouse, who suggested that attention was shifting from an emphasis on the *usefulness* of research findings to an obsession with their *truth value* or validity. Thus

> Without understanding why one course of action is better than another, we could prove by statistical treatment that it is. The vision is an enticing one: it suggests that we may make wise judgements without understanding what we are doing.
>
> (Stenhouse, 1978, p. 28)

As Stenhouse points out, all that is necessary in order to make a 'wise judgement' about practice is a knowledge of statistics and the research process. In other words, the ability to make judgements about research validity had replaced the ability to make judgements about practice. For Stenhouse, this was simply not good enough. Thus

> What I am trying to do is to encourage the feeling that all the statistics can be thrown out if they don't accord with the reality as you know it, and when you look at statistical results, somehow the thing to do is to end up not talking about standard deviations but talking about experience.
>
> (Stenhouse, 1985, p. 102)

The problem for Stenhouse and other educationalists was that the findings of research were being seen as of secondary importance to the method; that the quality criteria by which research was increasingly being judged was the internal and external validity of the study rather than the usefulness of the findings; that is, on its universal truth claims rather than on its local utility. The issue is not with truth *per se*; Stenhouse is not suggesting that the truth value of a research study is irrelevant, but rather that truth has come to be defined solely in terms of conforming to method, and that the criteria imposed upon researchers to ensure the internal and external validity of the study often inhibit the emancipatory quest for better health and social care. Because the status of evidence is determined largely by the research methods used to generate that evidence, there is far less scope in the classroom for informed discussion and debate about its impact on practice. Consequently, education for evidence-based practice centres increasingly around questions of research methodology rather than discussions about the suitability of research findings for practice and the problems and challenges involved in implementing findings. As Stenhouse suggests, we must ensure that we end up talking about experience rather than statistics.

Donald Schön echoed Stenhouse's plea to judge research according to its utility with his now well-known analogy:

> In the varied topography of professional practice, there is a high, hard ground overlooking a swamp. On the high ground, manageable problems lend themselves to solution through the application of research-based theory and technique. In the swampy lowland, messy, confusing problems defy technical solution. The irony of this situation is that the problems of the high ground tend to be relatively unimportant to individuals or society at large, however great their technical interest may be, while in the swamp lie the problems of greatest human concern. The practitioner must choose. Shall he remain on the high hard ground where he can resolve unimportant problems according to prevailing standards of rigor, or shall he descend to the swamp of important and non-rigorous inquiry?
>
> (Schön, 1987, p. 3)

This is, of course, a clear articulation of the conflict between the Enlightenment view of science as dealing with 'problems of human concern' and the post-Enlightenment view of science as rigorous and of technical rather than practical interest. Schön argues that these two aims are often incompatible, and that the practitioner must choose between the findings from rigorous but relatively unimportant research studies and non-rigorous, messy but relevant ones.

Unfortunately, as Schön suggests, we cannot have it both ways. Unbiased and objectively rigorous research comes at the cost of an insider perspective, which can result in a lack of interest and relevance. As Stenhouse (1981) points out, it is important that the researcher takes an *interest* in the outcome of her research, not only in the sense of being curious about the topic, but also in the sense of being personally involved and concerned about the outcome. Gadamer (1976) describes this interest as 'prejudice', which, as Koch (1994) notes, 'rather than getting in the way of research, makes research meaningful'. Similarly, universal and generalisable findings come at the cost of local context, and ultimately, the pursuit of truth and validity severely compromises relevance and application.

The existence of what a number of writers have referred to as the 'theory–practice gap' would suggest that academics in the health and social care professions are choosing rigour and truth over messiness and relevance; that practitioners are having difficulty in applying the rigorously conducted research studies disseminated from the ivory towers on the high hard ground to the messy uncertainty of everyday practice down in the swamp. There is a vicious circle at work here, where a creative approach to education is required in order to explore the messy world of practice, and yet the scientific quest for truth would appear to preclude any creative questioning of the so-called 'gold standard' research findings. There is no room for prejudice and subjectivity in the scientific application of evidence to practice. A refocusing on the Enlightenment's grand narrative of emancipation might sacrifice some of the objectivity and universal Truth of the findings, but would also go some way to addressing the problem of the theory–practice gap.

■ The general and the specific

I have argued above that, on the whole, academics in the health and social care disciplines have chosen truth rather than emancipation as the criterion of 'good' research. This, I have argued, has been a mistake and has contributed to the widening of the gap between academic theory and everyday practice. However, I believe that these academics also made a second and potentially even more damaging error in choosing the universal over the singular. Many of the first wave of health and social care researchers had backgrounds in the social sciences and were trained in the research methodologies of sociology and anthropology. And just as sociologists are generally concerned with developing theories about populations and societies, so these health and social care academics saw their aim as developing theories about the populations they were working with.

Whereas research findings about the behaviour of populations are very useful for informing public health initiatives or calculating the annual budget of an institution, they are of limited use to the health and social care practitioner in her everyday interactions with individual clients. As Max van Manen, writing about the practice of education, points out,

> Pedagogic situations are always unique. And so, what we need more of is theory not consisting of generalisations, which we then have difficulty in applying to concrete and ever-changing circumstances, but theory of the unique; that is, theory eminently suitable to deal with this particular pedagogic situation, this school, that child, or this class of youngsters.
>
> (van Manen, 1997, p. 155)

Or as Blake (1818/1927) put it, 'General knowledge is remote knowledge; it is in particulars that Wisdom consists and Happiness too.' However, the evidence-based practice movement appears to be taking us in the opposite direction, and almost every hierarchy of evidence on which practitioners are supposed to base their practice emphasises the importance of large-scale generalisable studies. Thus, in nursing, Evans has claimed that

> It can be argued that multicentre RCTs provide the best evidence for the effectiveness of an intervention because the results have been generated from a range of different populations, settings and circumstances. The findings from systematic reviews are generated in a similar manner, and so also provide rigorous evidence. As a result, the robustness and generalisability from both these approaches are better than what is generated by other research designs.
>
> (Evans, 2003, p. 81)

There is, however, a flaw in this logic. Whilst it is true that a large and carefully selected sample can lead to accurate predictions about the behaviour of the population from which it is drawn, the subsequent deduction from the general behaviour observed in that population to the behaviour of individual members holds only if each individual is identical to all the others. Whilst such an assumption might be relatively accurate for, say, responses to medications, the same cannot be said for responses to many (if not most) health and social care interventions. Different individuals not only respond differently to similar situations, but the same individual might well respond differently on different occasions, even when working with the same health and social care professional. As Sarvimaki (1988) says of nursing, it 'consists of interactions between unique individuals with unique experiences, and it always takes place in unique situations'. Hippocrates, the so-called 'father of modern medicine', knew this well, and is reported to have claimed that it is more important to know what sort of person has a disease than what sort of disease a person has. As Blake claimed above, wisdom is found in the particular rather than the general.

A shift in focus to the individual presents two challenges to the educationalist. Firstly, the subject matter must relate to individual cases rather than populations, for example by studying single case histories, novels, first-hand accounts by service users and providers, poetry and reflection-on-action. Secondly, the educational methods should focus on individual students and engage them in dialogues both with the material and with the educator. Once the remit of education moves beyond the transmission of facts and information, the curriculum is, of necessity, widened to encompass the psychological and affective domains in addition to (and perhaps more importantly than) the cognitive.

■ Conclusion

There is a tendency among theorists and practitioners who reject the 'hard science' approach to health and social care to argue for the 'artistry' of practice. In this chapter I have advocated an alternative solution by suggesting that we need to reclaim the original emancipatory aims of science as freeing us from pain, suffering and social inequality. In order to do so, we must challenge the currently dominant discourse in scientific research. Firstly, we must attempt to move away from the belief that the aim of research is to gain accurate and unsullied access to a universal Truth, and away from the obsession with rigour, validity and objectivity as the means to acquiring this Truth in its purest form. As Schön has pointed out, the most relevant research questions for practitioners can only be answered down in the swampy lowlands of practice itself, where messy questions require messy solutions. And secondly, we must get out of the habit of looking for single 'best' solutions to the problems of entire populations and refocus on unique interventions for unique individual therapeutic encounters.

In order for such a shift to take place, the current 'science of large numbers' which dominates evidence-based practice must be replaced with a 'science of the unique' (Rolfe and Gardner, 2005), with a focus on individual *persons* replacing the current obsession with groups of *people*. The current 'hard science' paradigm – with its implications of inflexible, unbending, rigid and rigorous adherence to the rules of method – is simply inappropriate for this reflexive focusing on the therapeutic encounter between individual persons.

I have argued that the hard science paradigm began in the academy when the dominant 'animating principle' of modern science shifted from emancipation to Truth. This shift quickly filtered down to health and social care practice, firstly with the research-based practice movement of the 1980s and latterly in a more 'hard science' version as evidence-based practice, where the quality of evidence is defined by a strict hierarchy with the randomised controlled trial at the top. It is tempting to think that, as educationalists, we have had nothing to do with this shift in the focus of health and social care research and practice. However, we should not forget that, as academics, we *are* (or should be) those very people who are determining what counts as 'good' evidence as well as having the responsibility for working with practitioners in addressing the problems of applying that evidence down in the swampy lowlands. The health and social care professions have a long tradition of innovation in education dating back several decades. The challenges involved in re-establishing these creative approaches to health and social care education must begin by challenging and reforming those very attitudes towards health and social care knowledge and knowledge generation that have contributed to their recent decline. The educational project of developing innovative curricula and learning interventions must therefore take place in conjunction with the equally important epistemological project of innovative research and practice development. Knowledge creation, communication and application must be seen as subsequent stages in the same process.

References

Blake, W. (1927). *Poems and Prophesies*. M. Plowman (ed.), London, Dent.
Brown, R.H. (1994). Reconstructing social theory after the postmodern critique. In H.W. Simons and M. Billig (eds) *After Postmodernism*, Sage, London.
Chomsky, N. (1988). *Language and the Problems of Knowledge*, MIT Press, Cambridge, Mass.
Comte, A. (1988). *Introduction to Positive Philosophy*, Hackett, Indianapolis.
Evans, D. (2003). Hierarchy of evidence: A framework for ranking evidence evaluating healthcare interventions. *Journal of Clinical Nursing*, **12**, 77–84.
Feynman, R.P. (1999). *The Pleasure of Finding Things Out*, Penguin, London.
Friedman, M. (1968). The methodology of positive economics. In M. Brodbeck (ed.) *Readings in the Philosophy of the Social Sciences*, MacMillan, London.
Gadamer, H.G. (1976). *Philosophical Hermeneutics*, University of California Press, California.
Galileo, (1967). *Dialogue Concerning Two Chief World Systems*, S. Drake (trans), University of California Press, California.
James, W. (1995). *Pragmatism*, Dover Publications, New York.
Koch, T. (1994). Establishing rigour in qualitative research: The decision trail, *Journal of Advanced Nursing*, **19**, 976–986.
Lyotard, J.-F. (1984). *The Postmodern Condition: A Report on Knowledge*, Manchester University Press, Manchester.
Lyotard, J.-F. (1992). *The Postmodern Explained to Children*, Turnaround, London.
MacIntyre, A. (1985). *After Virtue*, Duckworth, London.
Midgely, M. (2001). *Science and Poetry*, Routledge, London.
Payne, D. (1999). The knives are out for P2000, *Nursing Times*, **95**, 4, 14–15.
Phillips, R. (1994). The need for research-based midwifery practice, *British Journal of Midwifery*, **2**, 7, 335–338.
Popper, K. (1972). *Objective Knowledge: An Evolutionary Approach*, Clarendon Press, Oxford.
Pratt, V. (1978). *The Philosophy of the Social Sciences*, Routledge, London.
Readings, B. (1991). *Introducing Lyotard: Art and Politics*, Routledge, London.
Readings, B. (1996). *The University in Ruins*, Harvard University Press, Cambridge Mass.
Ridley, B.K. (2001). *On Science*, Routledge, London.
Rolfe, G. (2002). 'A lie that helps us see the truth': Research, truth and fiction in the helping professions, *Reflective Practice*, **3**, 1, 89–102.
Rolfe, G. and Gardner, L.D. (2005). Towards a nursing science of the unique: Evidence, reflexivity and the study of persons, *Journal of Research in Nursing*, **10**, 3, 297–310.
Sarvimaki, A. (1988). Nursing as a moral, practical, communicative and creative activity, *Journal of Advanced Nursing*, **13**, 462–467.
Schön, D. (1987). *Educating the Reflective Practitioner*, Jossey Bass, San Francisco.
Stenhouse, L. (1978). Case study and case records: Towards a contemporary history of education, *British Educational Research Journal*, **4**, 2, 21–39.
Stenhouse, L. (1981). What counts as research? *British Journal of Educational Studies*, **29**, 2, 103–114.

Stenhouse, L. (1985). The psycho-statistical paradigm and its limitations. In J. Ruddock and D. Hopkins (eds) *Research as a Basis for Teaching*, Heinemann, Oxford.

van Manen, M. (1997). *Researching Lived Experience*, Althouse Press, Ontario.

Wittgenstein, L. (1958). *Philosophical Investigations*, 2nd edition, G.E.M. Anscombe (trans), Basil Blackwell, Oxford.

Chapter 3

Patiently, telling the story

Phil Barker and Poppy Buchanan-Barker

■ Radical assumptions

This chapter embraces two simple assumptions about humanity and human behaviour. Both *arise from the roots* of our work in different human services, and both *go to the root* of the meaning of such services.

First, we believe that *all* that it means to *be a person* is found in story. Simply stated, all we are is our stories. We also believe that people deny this reality, or avoid facing it, by relating to people at some abstract level, using various typologies – for example, stereotypes, diagnostic types, personality types. This tactic allows them to avoid encountering the *actual* person. They relate instead to some romantic, disparaging or grossly oversimplified construction of the person, which fits their purpose.

■ Narratives and storytelling

Here we are addressing 'patient' stories and how the provision of care in any setting is influenced by the manner in which that story is heard. In some settings people are addressed with complete comfort as 'patients' – especially by nurses, doctors or dentists. However, social care professionals have, for generations, avoided the 'patient' title, preferring instead to talk of 'clients' or, more recently, users or consumers. We might assume these terms to be fairly neutral labels. However, they carry significant meanings, at least historically, especially in terms of the respective power of the parties involved.

In professional circles 'patient' means (simply) any 'person who receives medical attention'. This is a bland definition, since such attention could range from life-saving surgery to providing a repeat prescription for an antacid. The archaic definition – 'a person who suffers' – seems more telling, directing attention to the indefinable human experience (suffering), which makes the professional presence meaningful. However, the linguistic definition is more revealing: 'a noun or noun phrase identifying one that is *acted upon* or undergoes an action', suggesting the power relationship between the 'acted upon' *patient* and the professional doing the acting.

The term *client* derives from *cliens* (L), a member of the plebeian class in Ancient Rome, who lived under the protection of a *Patrician*. The power relationship was transparent. The *cliens* did things for the Patrician, gaining, in return, protection. In effect, the *cliens* was a *dependant*. People who need to use services as clients – for example, health, social care or the law – are similarly dependent: relying on the professional's authority, skill and commitment.

Over the past 30 years, organised attempts have been made to replace the use of the term 'patient' with that of 'client', 'consumer' or 'service user', especially in the mental health field. In part, these moves stem from the work of activists, unhappy with the power differential between the notions of 'patient' and 'professional', whether implied or actual. However, despite such concerns fretting, the 'patient' title often remains firmly embedded in 'health care language', and many physicians, in particular, resist vigorously any attempts to displace it (Neuberger and Tallis, 1999; Ritchie, Hayes and Ames, 2000).

■ The patient's story

Approaching his 38th birthday, Marc began to experience difficulty swallowing. He waited for it to pass. Over the next few months it seemed to wax and wane and his GP said it was 'probably nerves'. Within six months, swallowing had become much more difficult. Marc kept on working, also starting a second business from home. At times he felt weak. The GP advised that there was nothing wrong, but sent him for barium X-ray, which showed nothing of any significance. The GP was satisfied but Marc was struggling. Now both his legs had begun to swell below the knee. The GP diagnosed sarcoidosis. He had 'several patients in the practice with this condition'. Marc was worried as a website said it could be 'fatal'.

One day, walking his dog, he collapsed, and was rushed to hospital, where a pulmonary embolism was diagnosed. He recovered and went home on anticoagulants. The swallowing grew more problematic but the physician was concerned only with his blood. A haematologist called him in for some tests just before Christmas and decided to pass a 'scope', just to 'have a look-see'. On Christmas Eve, the haematologist came to his room wearing (as Marc recalled) a tie with Christmas decorations on it. He advised him that there was 'something pretty nasty' in his throat. In the first week of the New Year, he promised to get a surgeon to look at it properly. 'For now', he said 'you can stay here or go home. You decide.' Marc went home.

It was nasty. When Marc was unfit to travel a fortnight later the surgeon told Marc's family that it was 'beyond surgery. I doubt more than three months.' Marc persevered with radiotherapy and chemotherapy over the next six months, his patient journey peppered with hair loss, weight loss and considerable blood loss. He had two major haemorrhages at home and on one occasion the ambulance crew refused to move him. 'Being on the top floor, the stairs are too dangerous', they said, as his wife mopped blood from the floor and walls. Different GPs *now* paid home visits, but spoke mostly to his wife, as did the Macmillan nurses, who walked his dog, but shied away from talking to Marc other than in what he described as a 'daft, upbeat manner'. He died peacefully in a hospice ten months after the fateful Christmas.

■ **Personal space and impersonal distance**

How close we are allowed to get to people, when relating to them, varies across cultures (Williams, 2007). Hall (1966) popularised the notion of 'personal space' – the area that represents our 'domain' or territory. Like other animals, when this space is invaded, we feel uncomfortable, if not actually threatened.

Anglo-Europeans possess a characteristic *reserve* in which they tend to 'keep their distance', often contacting people only through ritualised 'handshakes'. The many different health care staff Marc encountered during his illness appeared to him to be typically 'Anglo-European'. Indeed, he put himself in this category, at least until he fell ill. Loath to talk about his feelings, hug people or make any obvious show of affection, he was not exactly aloof, but did appear emotionally 'cool'.

Illness, especially when life-threatening, changes people. Faced with the possibility that life might change – or might even be cut short – people take stock, of themselves and the meaning of their lives. Terry Eagleton (2007) dedicated his book *The Meaning of Life* to 'Oliver, who found the whole idea deeply embarrassing'. Marc, too, found such talk embarrassing until Life confronted him with 'meaning' and threatened its disappearance.

In talking about his experience of different doctors, nurses and the occasional social worker, Marc noted that although some were 'nice enough' others were 'hard work'. Even those whom he could relate to, however, 'kept their distance' and 'didn't really ask me anything about me'. There appears to be an invisible point at which 'personal space' blurs into interpersonal distance, an observation further discussed by McAndrew and Warne in Chapter 9.

Marc's doctors and nurses may not have been aware that they were 'standing back', but his animal sense detected this. He knew they were afraid of him. Of course, they had good enough reason, at least at the animal level, since Marc was *jinxed*. He was bad luck, reeking of ill-fortune, a harbinger of the death they all would face at some point.

However, at least in principle, all these professionals were trained to *relate*. Many would have completed 'counselling' courses and had experience of 'breaking bad news to patients' or their families. Yet, Marc still felt displaced, falling back on his wife and family as the 'only people who I can talk to or who will listen'. Perhaps his various carers had not yet come to terms with their own mortality (Barker and Buchanan-Barker, 2006).

■ The psychiatrist's story

The American psychoanalyst Harry Stack Sullivan was influential in his day but, according to his biographer, is now largely forgotten. The reasons are relevant to this chapter. From an Irish Catholic family, Sullivan (1953) became famous for his development of *Interpersonal Theory*. However, he lost the support of his colleagues, becoming the victim of gossip and slander. In Barton Evans' view, Sullivan's colleagues suspected him of being both a schizophrenic and a homosexual: 'Lester Haven stated that Sullivan was "at least twice acutely psychotic himself"' (Evans, 1996: 17); and 'the "clearly autobiographic" nature of Sullivan's writings proves his homosexuality' (p. 17). Up until the mid 1970s homosexuality was diagnosable as a psychiatric disorder, and was a major focus for psychoanalysis in the early part of the 20th century. Neither were psychiatrists too keen on one of their number 'going crazy', assuming that madness and professionalism did not mix. Sullivan's 'uncanny ability to empathize with the most troubled individuals' also disturbed his colleagues (Evans, 1996:17). For Sullivan, 'empathy' meant that by connecting with his own problems, he might better understand those of the 'patient'. His peers took a different view, believing that his *'emotional problems* . . . prevented him from taking the attitude, "There is the patient, whom I, a sounder person with special insights, shall treat"' (Evans, 1996:18).

Perhaps, unsurprisingly, Sullivan developed the concept of 'self esteem', which – 80 years later – is lodged in the vernacular. Given Sullivan's doubts about his own value and worth as person, if not as a psychiatrist, he was obviously keen to understand where these doubts emerged from, and how his 'esteem' might be bolstered.

Today, we talk with considerable ease about 'self esteem', 'self image' and various other 'self' concepts (Furedi, 2004). However, in coining the expression, Sullivan sought to explore himself and the people he was working with. Today, our language is awash with psychiatric and psychological jargon. It trips off the tongue, but does it convey any special understanding, or is it merely pretentious gobbledegook? A more worrying question is, Do professionals use Sullivan's 'self concepts' – and a host of other medical terms – to distance themselves from the 'patient', denying their own frailty in the process?

■ Problems of human living

In some areas of health care, such as mental health, the language problem appears even more problematic, especially where the original notions of 'illness' and 'disease' have been rendered almost meaningless. Tuberculosis is clearly a disease, with a physical pathology, but to what extent are the human problems associated with 'depression', for example, a function of a similar 'disease' process? Emotional and behavioural similarities may exist between different people described as 'suffering from depression', suggesting 'dysfunctions with characteristic forms' (Kutchins and Kirk, 1999; Szasz, 1996). However, such a view risks representing almost any behaviour perceived as 'problematic' as a function of 'disease': for example, reckless driving; poor handwriting; bad record-keeping; or late filing of income tax returns.

Harry Stack Sullivan is also remembered for coining the term 'problems in living', which he preferred to *psychopathology*. In Sullivan's view, the problems that people experienced privately – and exhibited publicly – were problems in living. They found it difficult to live with themselves, or to live with other people. Despite the flirtation with 'interpersonal' relations over the past 50 years by many health and social care professionals (Williams, 2007), the attraction of professional jargon, and overly complex forms of diagnostic classification, appears overpowering. In many areas of health care – from post-traumatic stress syndrome to 'multiple personality disorder' – people express their problems of human living, often in articulate, but plain, English, only to have this re-framed as one 'condition' or another.

Ultimately, health and social care professionals, must ask, 'how does this (e.g. condition, disorder, disability or state of affairs) cause or contribute to a problem in the living of your life?' In asking such a question, professionals must be willing to hear a 'story', which may make the attribution of a diagnosis appear simplistic, if not irrelevant. The purpose of health care is to help people live with or overcome their problems, not merely to label them. Sam Samociuk and Anne Lawton take this notion further in Chapter 5, which explores the use of simulated patients to increase the effectiveness of health and social care education.

■ Reclamation – Bring the story back to the surface

Across the estuary from our home in Scotland lies Dundee airport. Once submerged below the waterline, this land was drained over many years, and protected from further flooding by a sea wall. What once was out of sight and was useless was *transformed* into something of great value. This transformation was accomplished slowly, with great effort and skill, not to mention considerable risk to the people involved in undertaking it.

Water offers a fitting metaphor for the process of *reclamation* that is possible for those whose lives have been submerged by the experience of any form of illness or disability. In reclaiming their lives from the waters of 'illness', 'distress' or 'disability', people bring to the surface the person who was, to a large extent, lost from view. When people reclaim their lives, they undertake the lengthy, difficult and often threatening process of draining the effects of illness and disability from their lives, transforming something that once was thought to be both *meaningless* and *worthless* into something of great value if not priceless. All such reclamation is undertaken through the process of storytelling. By talking about their experiences, discussing them with others and especially 'being heard', people reclaim the personhood that has been submerged by illness and the *language* of illness. Being defined as a 'patient' is perhaps the most significant way that the person is submerged by professional language.

■ The alien paradox

When we cast the person as 'patient' or 'client' we cast them as some alien *Other*, which poses a threat to our emotional, if not physical, security. Madness is an 'other' experience – something beyond the pale. However, everyone who has ever enjoyed a good dream, especially a lucid one, or experienced a nightmare *knows* the particular madness popularly called psychosis. The psychotic process may be waking, and therefore different, but the form is identical.

Psychiatry, and to a large extent psychology, continues to view the people who become patients or clients in much the same way as anthropologists from 100 years ago: categorising, classifying, and ultimately stigmatizing their various features, ways of behaving, whether towards themselves or others. Within society at large, such 'objective', colonial, anthropology has been supplanted by a shared experience of social and cultural difference. Today we are more interested in what it means to *be* an Egyptian or a Scot, especially within a multicultural context.

However, in health and social care, diagnostic and classification systems continue to be used in a *limiting* way, reducing people like Marc to a condition or disease, with a person only loosely attached. Why can we not express interest in the person who is carrying, or even imagining, the pathological 'thing' that threatens them (literally) and us (metaphorically)? Professionals are tempted to relate primarily to the condition or illness, rather than the person with the illness experience, as this delimited relationship promises a degree of safety, where the professional can, through talking knowledgeably and acting expertly, can avoid addressing all the uncertainties that illness brings (see also McAndrew and Warne's discussion in Chapter 9).

If we *were* aliens – from outer space – we might find it easier to *engage* the person who is the 'patient': expressing curiosity as to their different mental, emotional or human states; bridging the gulf of illness or disability that separates us; fostering a sense of connectedness. Since the alien anthropologist (imagine the likeable ET from Spielberg's film) cannot express human empathy, he/she would be *curious* to know what 'being human' is like. Most professionals believe that they already know what the patient is experiencing, assuming that they are the 'sounder person with special insights', so highly valued by Sullivan's colleagues.

However, even as fellow humans we can never know, *exactly*, what others experience, even when the circumstances appear to mirror our own: for example, loss, pain, fear. However, if we talk with you, listening attentively to your story, exploring some of its meanings with you, we may discover in what way your story reflects our own and where it differs. Your story might make a splash, like a small stone, into the pool of our common humanity, causing ripples that extend further and further into our identity as separate beings. Those metaphorical ripples can be seen as signals of connection but also may be viewed as potential disturbance.

■ Human distress

If we are *health*-oriented (concerned with wholeness or completeness) we must focus on *how* a person *lives* his/her life, not just on limiting illness. This is as true for doctors and nurses as for social workers or other 'therapists'. However, we are not *making* them whole – they are whole already. When people are in great pain – whether physical or emotional – they are whole and complete. The story of their experience is whole and intact. It includes everything that they have ever been, *plus* the pain, which may be a new entry in the logbook of their life. This was a simple but profound fact of Marc's life. Marc's story is the whole story.

The professional infatuation with logging features, characteristics and behaviours led many professionals to construct lengthy 'holistic assessments' documenting everything from the person's favourite nail varnish to their preferred religious practice. Such catalogues miss the point. Wholeness is *oneness*. It is an *experience*, not a collection of life features or events. In aiming to be holistic we need only enquire into the person's *experience* to make contact (however superficial) with their oneness as a person. By asking people to *relate* experience, and all its attendant meanings, we begin to explore the abstract world of their personhood.

■ Dumb, ignorant, stupid questions

Commonly, people do not ask about others' experience, either because they believe they already know or because they don't want to know.

To become person-focused we have to remind ourselves that we could never know *all of it*, no matter how long we spend with the person. However, by listening attentively, we might become less ignorant. More importantly, in the telling of the story, the person will come to know himself/herself better. The year before her death, we asked our friend and mentor, Hilda Peplau, to summarise her work on interpersonal relations in a few sentences. Her answer was, 'people make themselves up as they talk', adding, 'I'm doing it now.'

Peplau's epithet, which we cannot find in any of her published works, is as profound as it is simple. There is no 'story' lying, in some pre-published form, within the recesses of our selfhood or psyche. There may be important memories, thoughts, feelings and other, much vaguer, ill-defined experiences, buried among the assorted dross of our 'life experience'. However, people must pick their way carefully through the clutter of accumulated experience to begin to build a story. Friends, family and especially professionals can help them explore the illness experience by asking damn, fool, silly questions. Ignorance is a virtue.

- What is it like to feel as if you are being followed?
- What is it like to feel that life is no longer worth living?
- What do you mean?
- What are you thinking right now?
- Talk to me!
- Help me understand.

All, stumbling around the key question 'what is it like to be you?'

■ Experts by experience

The concept of 'experts by experience' has entered the bureaucratic language of health and social care in the UK. For example, the *Commission for Social Care Inspection* defines 'experts by experience' as 'people of all ages, with different impairments and from diverse cultural backgrounds who have experience of using social care services' (www.csci.org.uk). However, as McAndrew and Warne argue in Chapter 9, why limit this 'expert' status to the 'user of services'? Why not simply accept that experience provides us all with, at least the potential, for expert status. Every mother who has given birth, every amputee who has lost a limb and every sightless person blinded in an accident has a special knowledge of their own experience. All they require to do is to organise the potentially disordered details of circumstance into a story, which might express the unique nature of their expert situation.

The alien anthropologist could help the person do this by expressing interest in what is special, different, unique, unusual, or simply 'odd' about this particular mother, amputee or sightless person? This is the *idiographic* approach first defined by Kant, where we try to understand things, which may well be accidental and subjective, and which may well not apply to any other situation. Such details set this person apart from all other persons.

Given this 'expert' status, we can, with some justification, sit at the person's feet, and be taught about their experience. Traditionally, professionals of every class believe (or pretend) that the person is ignorant, or has only a limited understanding of the illness situation. This belief provides the fundamental rationale for professional practice – patients need professionals, in the same way that the plebeian *cliens* needs the support of the Patrician.

The alien anthropologist adopts a different perspective, assuming that the person *is living with* the condition and, therefore, accumulating expert knowledge of how this – *living with* – is done. Professionals avoid most of these interesting questions, choosing instead to provide the patient with information about their illness, condition and so on. Although not without value, by definition such information represents no more than a rehashed, condensed, bowdlerised version of *other people's stories* about their experience of *this* condition; rather like an Egyptologist telling an Egyptian what it means to be descended from the Pharaohs, when it would make more sense to ask this particular Egyptian to tell us his particular meaning.

■ Recovering life – Accepting death

The concept of recovery has become popular in mental health in most Western countries, but risks becoming part of the slipshod language of health care bureaucracy. The original recovery dialogue emerged 70 years ago with the development of the 'buddy system' of Alcoholics Anonymous (AA). AA recognised that for any help to occur, *first* of all, the person had to *tell the story* of alcohol dependence, and its various personal and social effects. AA also recognised that the nexus of recovery lay in the intense collaboration between the simple, but difficult and often profound telling of the story, and its attendant hearing. That bond – made through human connection – provided the support the person needed to begin to chart the course of recovery.

Of course, since it had no 'method' or 'technique' to patent, no profit could be made from it. This explains, in part, the reluctance of professionals to recognise its obvious 'success'. Ironically, AA believed that alcoholism was an 'illness' deriving from some unspecified 'disease' process. They also believed that the person would always remain an 'alcoholic' – cure was not possible. However, by abstaining from alcohol, people could recover their lives. The 'alcoholic' within AA recognises that this critical part of the life story can never be erased and, more importantly, the practices associated with its creation should never be revisited. This is both intriguing and profound. The 'illness' cannot be cured, but the 'patient' can recover!

If Marc ever believed that his situation was hopeless, and that death was inevitable, this did not prevent him from 'carrying on living'. Perhaps he only accepted the challenges of radiotherapy and chemotherapy in an effort to postpone death. Or, he accepted these as means to continue living long enough to be able to accept death. In that sense, 'accepting death' was part of the recovery of his life.

■ Talk is cheap, but priceless

People, with all sorts of serious problems in living – from terminal cancer to alcoholism – find solace and often relief from their distress by talking with other 'sufferers', who are in the same boat (Davison, Pennebaker and Dickerson, 2000; Kyrouz, Humphreys and Loomis, 2002). These 'mutual support aid groups' are often described as a 'lifeline', in much the same way that the Samaritans phone service appears to help people stave off suicide. As in the original AA model, nothing more complicated than 'talking' and 'listening' is involved. There are no clinical formulations, no diagnosis and prognosis; just stories that unfold, slowly and often painfully, as people 'bear witness', exploring the lessons learned through suffering.

Perhaps patients find solace and support so easily in such groups, because the group, collectively, embraces wisdom not present in each person individually. In such groups they will avoid the 'incurable hopes of their friends', which Nightingale observed, when people try to 'cheer the sick by making light of their danger or exaggerating their probabilities of recovery', with the result that the patient 'feels isolated in the midst of friends' (Nightingale, cited by Downie, 2000:237). Such 'incurable hopes' are defences against the uncertainty of illness and can be found in professional as well as lay forms of 'comfort'. Nightingale also noted that although obituaries and medical reports often refer to 'unexpected' deaths, 'there was every reason to expect that A. would die, and he knew it; but he found it useless to insist upon his own knowledge to his friends . . . '(Downie, 2000:237). Perhaps all health and social care professionals need to reclaim the simple moral embraced by Nightingale's observations. As she said, often the patient needs little more than

> a single person to whom he could speak simply and openly, without pulling the string upon himself of this shower-bath of silly hopes and encouragements; to whom he could express his wishes and directions.
>
> (Downie, 2000:237)

The opportunity to talk honestly and openly about experience is the oxygen of story; the denial of such support is akin to drowning. Nightingale's moral completes the narrative loop, with which we opened this chapter. Although some of the language and theoretical concepts of the 'narrative approach' can appear intimidating (Bruner, 1994; Josselson, 1995; Crossley, 2000), the principles are simplicity itself. People deal with their life experience by constructing stories about those experiences and by listening to the stories of others. By exploring the 'narrative' that flows through the telling of the story, we discover how all human activity and experience is full of meaning, and make sense of complex psychological and philosophical concepts, such as 'self' and 'personhood', by discovering what these concepts mean for the individual storyteller. In an age when 'science' is so highly prized and our concepts of 'humanity' and 'selfhood' derive from often obscure, arcane theories, individual and collective storytelling serves as a necessary corrective. The universal fact of human existence is that people use stories to express the meaning of their lives and themselves; not logical arguments or psychological formulations.

Conclusion

The ailing 'patient' – whether hoping for recovery or awaiting death – needs care imbued with the empathic sensitivity Sullivan sought in the psychiatric clinic and which Nightingale appreciated in the Crimea. Patients need to be understood as people in unusual circumstances: struggling to make sense of their plight or trying to work out how best to live with pain, distress or debility. When health and social care professionals can provide the conditions necessary for a full and honest hearing of the patient's story, they may hear echoes of their own, and be reminded of their own frailty. This hearing will not save the patient, and may even engender more distress. Such is the nature of our storied lives. We have to relate the tale to move on to the next blank page. By teaching others about our experience, we 'make ourselves up, as we talk'.

References

Barker, P. and Buchanan-Barker, P. (2006) The psychological impact of serious illness. In J. Cooper. (ed.) *Stepping into Palliative Care: 1 Relationships and Responses.* Oxford: Radcliffe Publishing Ltd.

Bruner, J. S. (1994) The 'remembered' self. In U. Neisser and R. Fivush (eds.), *The Remembering Self: Construction and Accuracy in the Self-Narrative* (pp. 41–54). New York: Cambridge University Press.

Crossley, M. L. (2000) *Introducing Narrative Psychology: Self, Trauma, and the Construction of Meaning.* Buckingham, UK: Open University Press.

Davison, K. P., Pennebaker, J. W. and Dickerson, S. S. (2000) Who Talks?: The Social Psychology of Illness Support Groups. *American Psychologist* 55 (2), 205–217.

Downie, R. S. (ed.) (2000) Florence Nightingale: Notes on Nursing. *The Healing Arts: An Oxford Illustrated Anthology.* Oxford: Oxford University Press.

Eagleton, T. (2007) *The Meaning of Life.* Oxford: Oxford University Press.

Evans F. Barton (1996) *Henry Stack Sullivan: Interpersonal Theory and Psychotherapy*. New York, Routledge.

Furedi, F. (2004) *Therapy Culture: Cultivating Vulnerability in an Anxious Age*. London: Routledge.

Hall, Edward T. (1966). *The Hidden Dimension*. Anchor Books.

Josselson, R. (1995) Imaging the real: Empathy, narrative, and the dialogic self. In R. Josselson and A. Lieblich (eds.), *The Narrative Study of Lives* (Vol. 3, pp. 27–44) Thousand Oaks, CA: Sage.

Kutchins, H. and Kirk, S. (1999) *Making us Crazy: DSM, the Psychiatric Bible and the Creation of Mental Disorders*. London: Constable.

Kyrouz, E. M., Humphreys, K. and Loomis, C. (2002) A review of research on the effectiveness of self-help mutual aid groups. In B. J. White and E. J. Madara (eds.), *American Self-Help Clearinghouse Self-Help Group Sourcebook (7th edition)*. Cedar Knolls, New Jersey: St Claire Health Services.

Neuberger, J. and Tallis, R. (1999) Do we need a new word for patients? *British Medical Journal*, 318, 1756–1758.

Ritchie, C. W., Hayes, D. and Ames, D. J. (2000) Patient or client? The opinions of people attending a psychiatric clinic. *Psychiatric Bulletin*, 24, 447–450.

Sullivan, H. S. (1953) *Interpersonal Relations Theory of Psychiatry*. New York: Norton and Norton.

Szasz, T. S. (1996) *The Meaning of Mind: Language, Morality and Neuroscience*. London: Praeger.

Williams, C. (2007) *Therapeutic Interaction in Nursing*. Boston and London: Jones and Bartlett Publishers Inc.

Part 2

Educational Activities and Creative Approaches for Health and Social Care Education

Part 1 of the book set out the context for the book. Part 2 is made up of a series of eight chapters, each of which seeks to explore how creative approaches and/or the use of creative endeavours can be used to promote more effective learning and understanding. Amongst other approaches, these chapters provide examples of the use of literature, poetry, film and art in capturing and expressing the essence of experience, emotion and knowledge. Through these examples the reader is given the opportunity to recognise the parallel processes, involved between what occurs in the learning environment and that which occurs in practice, which involve valuing experience, holding and containing emotions and enabling the use of self to bridge the gap between knowledge and meaning.

Perhaps unusually for a book that has 'health and social care' in its title, the first chapter, Chapter 4, in Part 2 explores the development of a new worker in health care, that of the nurse practitioner. Perhaps even more challenging is that, amongst other aims, this chapter seeks to set out the need for ensuring the 'nurse' remains a visible part of this new and emergent role. However, setting these challenges aside for one moment, this chapter presents some of the difficulties educators have in drawing upon existing educational frameworks and approaches in terms of preparing new members of the health and social care workforce. Some of these challenges are familiar, the hegemony of the medical profession being just one example. In this chapter, Timothy Wand and Brenda Happell promote the use of case studies as a way of bridging the gap between traditional and contemporary pedagogies, and this approach is evident in other chapters in Part 2. The theme of attending to new educational demands in different ways is built upon in Chapter 5. Here Sam Samociuk and Anne Lawton describe the challenges and successes of bringing into the classroom a range of simulated patients, who, using varies case study plots, are able to provide students with different learning opportunities in exploring the relationship between theory and practice. This is a discourse that is approached in a different way in Chapter 6, where Marie Crowe takes the reader through a carefully constructed case study in her exploration of psychodynamic and discursive approaches that can be used in sense-making. The case study is brought alive in Chapter 7, where Brenda Happell and Cath Roper share their work in developing the concept of the consumer academic in Australia. As in Chapter 5, a stimulating mixture of practical and inspirational experiences is discussed, with real-life challenges for teachers, students and institutions highlighted. In Chapter 8, a range of equally challenging approaches are discussed by Ann Gallagher and Andrew McKie in describing and discussing the work they have been engaged in which draws upon poetry and literature as the learning medium. Likewise, in Chapter 9, drawing upon their own experience in two different universities, Sue McAndrew and Tony Warne explore how involving students in hands-on painting can be used to enable students to deal with complex and often taboo areas of health and social care. The way in which popular culture, and in particular films, deals with such issues is the subject of Chapter 10. Here Gary Morris sets out a fascinating and rich analysis of the wealth of learning opportunities there might be in harnessing popular culture in this way, particularly where such use involves very familiar celebrities. Finally in Part 2, in Chapter 11, the reader is given the opportunity to see how many of these ideas can be brought together in an approach called Transformative Learning. Margaret McAllister explores this concept in a way that is representative of the meta–case study. That is, an account that recognises the need for new ways of thinking on the part of the teacher, the use of the familiar as a prompt for exploration for the student, and the use of the sometimes strange and unfamiliar to promote debate, discussion and change in thinking.

Whilst we are sure there will be elements in each of these chapters that you are also familiar with, we hope that in reading the ambitious, challenging and stimulating accounts that make up Part 2 of this book, the potential for being creative is revealed.

Chapter 4

Emphasising the 'nurse' in nurse practitioner: Challenges for educational preparation

Timothy Wand and Brenda Happell

■ Introduction

The Nurse Practitioner (NP) role is an exciting dynamic area of advanced nursing practice in contemporary health care. Emerging in the US in the mid-1960s, the NP role is now also established in Canada, the UK, Ireland, parts of Europe and Asia, Australia and New Zealand. It is now estimated that up to 40 countries worldwide have initiated NP programmes or are working towards this (Middleton et al., 2007).

As clinical experts with commensurate formal education at master's level or beyond, NPs are able to make complex decisions about what care and treatment is required. Authorisation as an NP also typically enables the nurse to prescribe and administer certain medications related to their specialty area, to initiate focused diagnostic investigations such as pathology tests and medical imaging (Wand & White, 2007a). The NP title is protected by state or national legislation in the US, Canada, Ireland, New Zealand and Australia.

Another challenge associated with NP preparation and practice is ensuring that qualities unique to nursing are maintained; the danger being that NPs may become more like medical practitioners, with the prescription of medication, ordering of diagnostic tests and other roles traditionally associated with medicine becoming the primary focus of practice.

Browne and Tarlier (2008) stated that valuing NPs primarily for their physician replacement value has proven problematic for the sustainability of the NP. This contributed to the demise of the NP movement in Canada in

51

the 1970s. Instead, Browne and Tarlier propose that ensuring NP role sustainability rests on recognising the value-added component of NP practice. They emphasise the social justice aspects of the role in the context of illness; incorporating treatment, health promotion and prevention services, and examining how discriminatory practices constrain people's access to health services.

Any new professional role is generally accompanied by a degree of uncertainty. The NP role is particularly challenging because of the expansion of functions into the practice domain of medicine. Medical practitioners are likely to feel a degree of boundary violation that nurses are encroaching on their territory and may therefore be reluctant to work collaboratively with NPs. Nursing colleagues may be uncertain and uncomfortable with the NP role and could possibly feel inadequate in comparison with NPs. Furthermore, role confusion between NPs and medical practitioners may emerge. For example, nurses may be unsure who they should consult with regarding medication issues. Similarly, allied health professions may be unclear as to the role of the NP. There is not likely to be an easy solution, but part of educating NP should also address this issue of role clarity.

An important aim of this chapter is to locate NP roles very firmly within the discipline of nursing, and to consider the implications of this from an educational perspective. More specifically, it is intended that the content of this chapter will address the following:

- A background to nurse practitioner roles.
- Appreciating the nursing perspective of nurse practitioners.
- Educating nurse practitioners: Challenges and opportunities.
- Making a difference: A mental health nurse practitioner in the emergency department.
- Creative approaches to the education of nurse practitioners.

■ Background

The introduction of NP roles has been largely welcomed by the nursing profession as an attractive clinically based career path that may encourage nurses to remain within the profession rather than seeking more fulfilling jobs elsewhere (Clinton & Hazelton, 2000). Clearly, however, NPs fit within a broader political and economic context that do and will continue to influence and impact on practice. The history of NP roles has been extensively described in the literature (Dunphy, Youngkin & Smith, 2004). It is not the aim of this chapter to reiterate or expand this discussion; however, a brief overview of the developing impetus and focus for NP roles provides a useful background.

In the US and Canada, the NP role developed in response to a shortage of medical officers (Torn & McNichol, 1996; Pearson & Peels, 2002). This was particularly apparent in rural areas, and suburbs perceived as undesirable because of low socio-economic status or higher incidence of illnesses. NPs were subsequently introduced to address apparent health care inequities. Despite the perception of a physician replacement quality to the implementation of NPs in the US, research on NP practice cited by Brown and Waybrant (1988) identified that the acquisition of medically oriented functions did not diminish NP activity in more traditional areas of nursing. The research at that time highlighted a specific emphasis in NP practice on health promotion, disease prevention and disease management, support, understanding, counselling, health education, health maintenance and a holistic approach to the client (Brown & Waybrant, 1988). The successful implementation of NP models in the US influenced the development of these roles in the UK (Elsom, Happell & Manias, 2005).

■ Appreciating the nursing perspective of nurse practitioners

Pearson and Peels (2002) stated that the raison d'être for the NP is to meet clients' needs in populations that are underserved. Nurses working in specific contexts may therefore need to extend their role to meet the health care needs of particular patient groups. However, this need not detract from the caring aspect of nursing that concentrates on humanising the health system at the point of contact through health teaching and the provision of physical, emotional and psychological support.

Gardner et al. (2006) emphasised that a 'nursing model' should be the core tenet in the preparation for NP practice, and acknowledge the centrality of clinical, self-directed learning as an essential characteristic of NP educational preparation. This incorporates consideration of the diverse specialty streams and clinical environments in which NPs work and the need for a range of skills to ensure professional and public safety.

The progression of NP roles has frequently been constrained my medical groups expressing concerns that NPs are an attempt to substitute nurses for medical officers (Pearson & Peels, 2002). However, reports and evaluations from the available mental health nursing literature, for example, consistently maintain that the mental health NP (MHNP) is complementary to specialised medical roles. There is emphasis placed on MHNPs retaining and cultivating the humanistic qualities of nursing in order to ensure that the public continue to experience the distinct therapeutic benefits of advanced mental health nursing practice (Fisher, 2005; Elsom, Happell & Manias, 2005; Wand & Fisher, 2006; Wortans, Happell & Johnston, 2006; Wand & White, 2007a).

■ Educating nurse practitioners: Challenges and opportunities

Despite the importance attributed to NP roles and their strong position internationally, there is a paucity of research addressing the educational preparation of NPs. This would appear to reflect a lack of consistency in educational standards and approach (Gardner et al., 2006). Gardner et al. (2006) undertook a detailed investigation of NP curricula in Australia and New Zealand. Their findings revealed marked inconsistency in a number of areas including programme content. Only 3 content areas were found in all 14 courses: pharmacology, research, and assessment and diagnosis. Additional areas found common to many included anatomy and physiology; professional nursing practice; scope of practice; clinical leadership; society, law and ethics; and cultural aspects of nursing practice. Most courses also provided scope for students to concentrate on a specific area of specialty practice.

It is an issue of some concern that of the three areas common to all, two are concerned with medical practice, and the remaining one pertains to research. This is not to suggest that these three areas are not all important for and relevant to NP practice. However, this clearly identifies a challenge for the education of NPs in these two countries and indeed internationally. If NPs are to make a positive contribution to health care across a broad range of practice settings in the interests of those who use services, they must clearly continue to identify and be identified as nurses. Nursing practice and the unique contribution of nurses must be an obvious feature of all NP education programmes.

Browne and Tarlier (2008) promoted educational strategies for the NP that concentrate on a critical analysis of how, for example, does social positioning mediate access to health services or how certain policies constrain access to health care in conjunction with education on the biomedical basis for disease and treatment. This would enhance the capacity for NPs to respond to forms of social suffering that result from inequities.

Gardner et al. (2006) asserted that structured pedagogical approaches of learning are inadequate for NP education. These authors advocated a 'capability approach' to the learning process, which incorporates the flexibility to respond to specific, self-identified learning needs of students. Becoming capable requires different learning experiences from becoming competent. Capable practitioners are those who know how to learn, are creative, have a high degree of self efficacy, are able to apply competencies in novel and familiar situations and work well with others (Gardner et al., 2006).

In contrast with the problem-based approach espoused by the medical model, nursing authors are now considering solution-focused strategies to inform clinical practice and research particularly in mental health (McAllister, 2003; Stevenson Jackson & Barker, 2003; Hosany et al., 2007;

Lamprecht et al., 2007; Walsh & Moss, 2007; Ferraz & Wellman, 2008; McAllister et al., 2008). In addition to mental health, solution-focused approaches in nursing have been described in a variety of practice domains such as early parenting and working with children and families (Carter, 2007; Rowe & Barnes, 2007), learning disabilities (Musker, 2007), youth work (McAllister, 2007), acute medical care (Henderson, 2007), chronic illness (Gardner & Gardner, 2007) and dementia care (Adams & Moyle, 2007). Solution-focused nursing provides a much needed alternative for nurses who are aiming to work with clients to restore and maintain health and well-being (McAllister, 2003). A solution orientation concentrates on what is going right with an individual or group and aims to maximise human potential through engagement in order to build on personal resilience and strengths, achievements and capacity (McAllister, 2007).

McAllister (2003) maintained that a problem focus may be useful for disciplines such as medicine, but not so useful for nursing, which has a strong focus on human relationships and identifying strengths and abilities in individuals. If nursing students are encouraged to be problem finders and solvers, then they may be unable to function in any other capacity. Intervening and taking control prematurely, acting as the expert, offering only a passive role to patients, ignoring personal strengths and abilities and fostering an illness mentality are all aspects of health care that need to be challenged (McAllister, 2003).

By illustration, Walsh et al. (2008) adopted solution-focused strategies to resolving complex clinical practice issues through a process they call 'puzzling practice'. They proposed that unlike problems, puzzles imply a shared enterprise with no attribution of blame. Solutions to puzzles can be developed one piece at a time and often require innovative and creative approaches. Walsh and colleagues contended that this is much more than a semantic exercise. This approach is based on the premise that problem-based ways of working can interfere with the generation of effective solutions and that understanding the cause of the problem is not necessarily associated with resolving it. Puzzling can be part of a genre of structured action learning and action change that can have a dramatic effect on engagement and solution generation. Cognitive mechanisms such as re-framing, re-languaging, re-imaging and re-imagining practice can make a difference to the ways in which clinical issues are understood and action generated in relation to them.

In this instance, a 'puzzle group' of eight specialist nurses meet monthly to work through a difficult clinical situation. A clinical example is used from the perspective of a cardiac rehabilitation nurse specialist. This clinician was experiencing difficulties in complying with a protocol that required her to call each patient following a myocardial infarction four times post discharge over a number of weeks. Together, the puzzle group were able to assist the nurse to formulate a puzzle statement, visualize a range of possible solutions and devise an action plan to be systematically implemented over a couple of months. Walsh et al. believed that this approach can be applied with good effect by individuals and groups in many contexts and clinical settings (Walsh et al., 2008).

☐ Reflective exercise

List what you believe are the essential skills, knowledge and attitudes that should be reflected in curricula for NP practice and from your list consider the following:

- What would be equally applicable to nurses in roles other than NPs?
- What would be more commonly attributed to medical practitioners?
- From your own experience with NP curricula, which do you believe are most strongly reflected?
- What principles should underpin curriculum development to ensure these are equally reflected?

The first step in designing educational programmes for NP should reflect the vision for the role, in particular the health care needs the position is designed to meet and deliver. In simple terms, what do we want NP to do? How do we think they should be different from other members of the health care team? What particular characteristics of the role do we value? The following section provides an overview of a specialist MHNP in the emergency department (ED) of a general hospital. In articulating the role and identifying the unique contribution it provides to health care we can move closer to determining some essential content for NP curricula.

■ Making a difference: A mental health nurse practitioner in the emergency department

Due to mainstreaming mental health services, there has been a significant increase in the prevalence of people experiencing a mental illness within the general health care system in Australia (Happell & Platania-Phung, 2005). Consequently, the ED has become a major point from which mental health services are accessed (Wand & White, 2007b). General hospital staff therefore have frequent contact with people with significant mental health needs (Sinclair et al., 2006). Research findings indicate that emergency nurses often lack the expertise, motivation and confidence to adequately address these mental health needs (Gillette, Bucknell & Meegan, 1996; Heslop, Elsom & Parker, 2000; Wand & Happell, 2001; Clarke, Dusome & Hughes, 2007; Kerrison & Chapman, 2007).

The ED is an ideal setting for an MHNP. This role can bridge the gap between mental and physical health services by providing expertise and support to ED staff and consumers of mental health services (Wand, 2004). The ED therefore provides an ideal setting to articulate the role and contribution of the NP, and to consider the importance of educational preparation.

Recognition of the important contribution an NP could make in the emergency setting is not a new concept. Torn and McNichol (1996) argued that an NP with expertise in mental health could improve access to specialist care for clients and improve awareness of mental health issues amongst general hospital staff. Clinton and Hazelton (2000) also envisaged the MHNP working in the ED as a role that could make a significant contribution in supporting nurses and medical staff where mental health presentations are a growing issue. This vision was supported by the findings of an Australian study (Gardner & Gardner, 2005). The inclusion of an MHNP to provide consultation–liaison services to the general hospital and the ED resulted in improved access and reduced waiting times.

Wand and Fisher (2006) described the introduction of an MHNP role at the Royal Prince Alfred Hospital (RPAH) in Sydney, Australia. The role developed on the strength of a successful pilot (Wand & Happell, 2001). The primary function of the MHNP concerns the provision of prompt assessment, therapeutic intervention and coordination of care for people presenting with a range of mental health difficulties (Wand, 2004). This MHNP position is based on a collaborative relationship between the Area Mental Health Service and the RPAH and founded on the principles of mental health liaison nursing (MHLN) described by Roberts (1997; 2002). The positive outcomes associated with the MHLN role based in the ED have been identified from a number of evaluation reports worldwide. High levels of ED staff and consumer satisfaction have been documented especially in relation to reduced waiting times, on-site access to expert mental health assessment, therapeutic intervention, coordination of care and raised mental health awareness among ED staff (Gillette, Bucknell & Meegan, 1996; Brendon & Reet, 2000; Callaghan et al., 2001; Wand & Happell, 2001; Hughes & Clarke, 2002; McDonough et al., 2004; Wand, 2004; Clarke et al., 2005; Sinclair et al., 2006; Eales, Callahan & Johnson, 2006; Wand & Schaecken, 2006).

■ Examples from practice: Personal reflections of the nurse practitioner role

To place the NP role in a broader context, the following are some personal reflections on the development and current status of the role as experienced by one of the authors:

Over the four years that I have been employed in the capacity of nurse practitioner I have noticed a shift in my practice, and the attitude of colleagues I work with has also changed. It has been gratifying to experience the recognition and positive regard from nursing colleagues. As medical colleagues become more familiar with the NP role they too are able to perceive a difference and appreciate the clinical availability and specialised nursing expertise inherent in the role. I have been fortunate to find myself in an environment where I am supported in my NP role development at both the clinical and administrative level. Recently the administration acknowledged the change in my practice by establishing a nurse consultant position to complement my NP role.

I have always seen myself primarily as a clinician, which is why I was attracted to the NP role. Nurse Practitioners see patients, and that is what I spend most of my working day doing. I have assumed more of a total care function for many of the patients I see through the ED; the initial assessment, intervention, health education and promotion, medication prescribing, discharge, referral, follow-up. Becoming an NP has enhanced my ability to assume a holistic approach. The NP possesses the required skills and characteristics for the delivery of specialised primary care. Of course I still often rely on the contributions and advice of ED nursing and medical staff as well as colleagues in psychiatry. You are still very much a part of a team, but the work is now that bit more autonomous and rewarding.

■ The nurse practitioner in action

Case studies are commonly used as a tool to facilitate nursing education. Case studies provide the opportunity to move beyond theoretical principles and encourage critical thinking and problem-solving skills (DeSanto-Madeya, 2007). Given some of the issues discussed in this chapter, case studies can have particular benefits for the education of NP. For example, this approach provides a framework to encourage students to maintain a strong focus on nursing to ensure this is not lost with the expansion of their practice. In this section we present three case studies based on one of the authors' practice. These case studies are based on real people and real issues. However, the names and some of the details have been changed to protect the privacy of the people involved. These case studies have deliberately been presented in the first person to more accurately and personally portray the interaction between the NP and the client and hopefully reflect the unique contribution of nursing. The case studies are followed by reflective exercises to demonstrate how they might be used as an educational tool.

Case study – Anita, a solution-focused approach

Anita presented to the ED one evening in a distressed state, accompanied by her husband Joshua, reporting a three-week history of vertigo that had been constant over the previous five days. Anita and Joshua had been involved in a bus accident while on holiday in Southeast Asia several months prior to this presentation. Anita had required a brief hospital stay after the accident and sustained a back injury for which she was receiving regular physiotherapy. Since the accident Anita had experienced severe vertigo accompanied by a fear that she would either faint or fall over. She had seen her GP on a number of occasions, who had performed numerous medical tests and investigations including a CT and MRI scan.

Anita was seen by an ED registrar. She disclosed that she also had a history of anxiety, panic and depressive symptoms and agreed that she was very distressed by her back pain and vertigo. Anita felt certain that an underlying physical cause accounted for her symptoms. She agreed to stay in the ED overnight and was amenable to speaking with the ED MHNP in the morning.

When I saw Anita she was obviously distressed. On discussing her circumstances, Anita agreed that anxiety and panic over her symptoms were contributing to her distress; however, she maintained that her condition must have a physiological connection to the accident in Southeast Asia. I did not challenge this perception but invited her back to the ED to see me in my outpatient service. Anita contacted me a few days later and arranged an appointment.

In solution-focused brief therapy (SFBT) the central assumptions are that the goals for therapy are chosen by the client and that clients themselves have resources which they will use in making changes. A detailed history is not essential. Sufficient improvement is often achieved in three to five sessions and approximately 25 per cent of clients require only one session. However, like other psychotherapies, long-standing problems are less responsive to intervention (Macdonald, 2007).

There are several specific and broad strategies used in SFBT such as scaling, exploring for exceptions, a technique called the miracle question, and providing compliments and end-of-session feedback. In addition to this, the solution-focused practitioner expresses a genuine interest in the client and the client's own frame of reference, drawing on and amplifying client strengths as the expert of their own experience.

Anita reported to me that her ongoing vertigo was causing high levels of mental distress. She reiterated her belief that a physical cause must be underlying her state, claiming that her symptoms couldn't possibly be accounted for by anxiety and panic alone. Recently, Anita had been socialising less due to her symptoms and stated that Joshua was becoming frustrated with her. Anita was still able to get to sleep easily and maintain her job as an occupational therapist in an acute mental health unit. She had also recently taken on some additional work lecturing to undergraduate students at the university. Despite the stress of her work environment and the extra university work, Anita still managed to get out of the house each day, albeit with great difficulty.

Through exploration of her situation, Anita recognised that while the mornings were very hard for her, the anxiety and panic symptoms were less prominent once she was at work or university. Anita had also noticed that she usually felt better generally when regularly attending yoga classes or running on the treadmill at the gym. She had recently stopped these activities due to her fear that she might lose balance or faint in public.

My first response was to acknowledge how difficult it must be for Anita to tolerate and manage her symptoms. I asked Anita to place herself on a scale from 1 to 10 in terms of how well she thought she was able to control her anxiety and panic symptoms, where 1 is 'not at all' and 10 is 'complete control'. Anita gave herself a 4. We first discussed how she was at 4 and not lower on the scale. I then asked Anita to consider what would need to change for her to move one or two points up the scale.

Anita and I explored how she managed to go to work and attend the university – How do you do that? – and what she was actually doing to 'keep it together' during that time. Anita was able to reflect on and articulate the mental skills and strategies that she was using to get herself out of the house in the morning and to maintain her composure throughout her workday. This process assisted Anita to recognise what she was already doing to manage her symptoms and how we could use this information to build on further progress.

Over three sessions Anita and I were able to obtain a detailed picture of what might help to improve her ability to manage her symptoms. Anita returned to yoga classes and the gym. She practised the self-talk and breathing techniques that usually assist individuals to enhance control over their anxiety and panic symptoms. By the third session Anita had placed herself at 6 on the 'controlling her symptoms' scale. She was also able to envisage moving further up the scale and identified what would be different (and what she would then be doing differently) to indicate that she had reached a higher point on the scale.

☐ *Reflective exercise*

- Brainstorm your immediate response to this scenario.
- Do you consider the interactions between Tim and Anita were beneficial for Anita?
- Identify the aspects of the relationship you consider were beneficial or not beneficial for Anita.
- How do you feel Anita's experience with the ED may have differed if she was seen by

  o An emergency nurse?
  o An emergency physician?
  o A psychiatrist?
  o A mental health nurse without NP status?

- How do you feel being an NP contributed to Tim's management of Anita's situation?
- To what extent do you think Tim's background and role as a nurse contributed to this relationship?

Case study – Sebastian

Sebastian presented to the ED via ambulance with chest pain and shortness of breath. Sebastian was a student at the local university. He was seated in front of a computer working on his thesis when he suddenly developed the symptoms. Medical examination and investigations indicated no cardiac involvement and the ED medical officer suggested to Sebastian that his presentation may be related to mental stress. Sebastian agreed and the medical officer referred him to me.

Sebastian told me that he had been working long hours on his thesis and felt anxious and mentally drained. He had been to his GP and was prescribed paroxetine but thought that it had only made him feel worse. Sebastian found meeting his family, academic and part-time work commitments exhausting (he has a wife and a small child). He and his wife were from overseas and had no family and only few supports locally. Sebastian had previously engaged in regular exercise but had now ceased because he had no time to spare. He had not had any time off from work or studies in over two years.

I spoke to Sebastian about the physical and mental symptoms associated with panic and discussed some strategies for symptom management. I also gave him some information sheets to take home and read. I explained to Sebastian that the anti-depressant he was prescribed might have contributed to his recent symptoms. Together, we also established that regular exercise had previously been a mechanism for Sebastian to maintain his general health and that stopping this could have influenced the onset of his anxiety and panic.

Sebastian was reluctant to continue with the anti-depressant medication preferring to address his problem from a psychological perspective. He agreed for me to speak with his GP about ceasing the anti-depressant and seeing a clinical psychologist. I phoned the GP, who agreed that a psychologist would be beneficial for Sebastian and was happy to arrange a referral. I gave Sebastian numbers for psychologists in the area near where he lived and wrote a discharge letter for him to take to the GP and the psychologist.

Authorisation as an NP in Australia formalizes the right to refer to specialists; however, in a case like this it is important for the primary physician to be maintained as the conduit for ongoing care. Some months later I received an email from Sebastian saying that he still had occasional symptoms but the psychology service had been helpful. He had resumed exercising and had recently returned from a holiday with his family to visit relatives overseas.

☐ *Reflective exercise*

- Again we ask you to consider how Sebastian's experience of ED treatment may have been different under the care of a medical officer or a nurse.
- What aspects of the care and treatment Tim provided were particularly noteworthy?
- How do you think that Tim contributed to Sebastian's overall sense of health and well-being?

One of the particularly interesting features of Sebastian's case is that Tim encouraged and advocated for alternatives to traditional medical treatment for Sebastian. He did this, firstly, by supporting his decision to see a psychologist in preference to continuing with his anti-depressant medication and, secondly, by encouraging Sebastian to resume regular exercise as an important determinant of his health and overall well-being. It is unlikely that such a comprehensive approach could be provided by any other health professional.

Case study – Selim

Selim presented overnight requesting a depot injection of anti-psychotic medication. He told the ED medical officer that he usually has a fortnightly injection. In the past few days he had moved from a suburban boarding house where he had lived for many years and was now living in an inner city men's refuge. Selim stated that he had moved out of the boarding house because another resident was continually threatening him. In the morning I was asked to see Selim. I had met him previously.

Selim is from a Middle Eastern background with reasonable English, though he has no family or friends in Australia. He has a long history of mental illness and has had numerous previous admissions to mental health units in the area. He is a placid man with no previous history of drug or alcohol abuse. Selim did not appear to be in any distress and reported no acute psychotic symptoms. He was happy to stay at the refuge for the time being. Selim was unsure of the type of injection or the usual dose, but stated it had been over two weeks since he last received it. He was previously receiving his depot injection from a GP who came to the boarding house. He no longer had any contact with the community mental health team (CMHT) and stated that no arrangements were made for his follow-up injections or mental health care when he left the boarding house.

I arranged a discharge summary from Selim's last admission, which had only been three months prior. The discharge summary confirmed that he was on zuclopenthixol decanoate 200mg fortnightly. I was then able to prescribe and administer the injection myself. This ability to prescribe and administer medication saves valuable time in the ED setting. The CMHT near to the men's refuge has a clinic for depot injections and I contacted them regarding follow-up injections and general support for Selim. I faxed over the ED notes and a copy of the discharge summary and treatment sheet. I then spoke to a welfare officer at the refuge. The refuge is run by a charity organization that has access to long-term accommodation. The welfare officer stated that he would be happy to meet with Selim and discuss options for community housing. I gave Selim my details and the contact details and location of the CMHT where he could go for his injection and mental health needs.

☐ *Reflective exercise*

- What are some of the problems in providing health care to people with a long-term mental illness that become evident through Selim's situation?
- How was Tim able to address these problems?

■ Implications for educating nurse practitioners

It is not within the scope of this chapter to develop an NP curriculum in even a skeletal form. However, exploring the introduction of an NP role in a general hospital ED has provided the opportunity to consider some of the features of this role that should underpin curriculum development and implementation. These include the following:

- The unique contribution of nursing to NP roles: This should be both explicit and pervasive throughout the curriculum. While skill and expertise in the diagnosis, assessment and medication prescription is crucial, the nursing perspective needs to underpin all aspects of the theoretical programme.
- Communication skills, with particular emphasis on the ability to relate sensitively to the distressed person in order to elicit relevant information while managing and containing stress and anxiety.
- Health education: The NP has a crucial role in providing information, both verbal and written. While it may be assumed that nurses and therefore NPs are effectively able to perform as an educator, this role is too important to be left to chance. NP curricula should therefore include a focus on health education and health promotion, particularly (but not exclusively) in relation to the following areas:

  o Education about specific illnesses.
  o Medications including desired and unwanted effects.
  o The importance of general health and well-being.
  o Alternatives to medical approaches to overcoming illness and achieving health.

- Consumer perspective: The research and broader literature around NP roles continually reveal a high level of satisfaction with NP because the nature of the relationship between NP and the service user is qualitatively different to that of other relationships in the health sector. The role of the NP is to enhance continuity of care and, as client advocate, must also be a feature of NP curricula.

The use of case studies and other creative approaches will assist future NPs to focus practice on the needs of people requiring care, combining the long-standing nursing background with the newly acquired expanded skills to become an important and unique part of contemporary health care delivery. Case studies provide the opportunity to move beyond the theoretical to consider the health care needs of people as individuals rather than as collections of symptoms to be treated.

■ Conclusion

Nurse practitioners are likely to become a strong part of the health care system of the future. There is now considerable evidence to support the quality of and satisfaction with the care provided by NP. Importantly, NPs are not substitute doctors and the important contribution that nursing brings to this role must be maintained. The educational preparation of NPs is charged with the responsibility of ensuring that nursing remains a strong focus and is visibly apparent within the curricula. Developing NP curricula requires careful consideration and a vision for the NP role. Creative strategies such as case studies and reflective practice will help to keep the 'nurse' firmly entrenched in the nurse practitioner.

References

Adams, T., & Moyle, W. (2007). Transitions in aging: A focus on dementia care nursing. In M. McAllister (ed.) *Solution Focused Nursing: Rethinking Practice.* Palgrave: Hampshire, UK, pp. 154–162.

Brendon, S., & Reet, M. (2000). Establishing a mental health nurse service: Lessons for the future. *Nursing Standard* 14 (17), 43–47.

Brown, M. A., & Waybrant, K. M. (1988) Health promotion, education, counselling, and coordination in primary health care nursing. *Public Health Nursing* 5 (1), 16–23.

Browne, A. J., & Tarlier, D. (2008). Examining the potential for nurse practitioners from a critical social justice perspective. *Nursing Inquiry* 15 (2), 83–93.

Callaghan, P., Eales, S., Leigh, L., Smith, A., & Nichols, J. (2001). Characteristics of an accident and emergency liaison mental health service in east London. *Journal of Advanced Nursing* 35 (6), 812–818.

Carter, B. (2007). Working it out together: Being solution-focused in the way we nurse with children and their families. In M. McAllister (ed.) *Solution Focused Nursing: Rethinking Practice.* Palgrave: Hampshire, UK, pp. 63–76.

Clarke, D. E., Dusome, D., & Hughes, L. (2007). The emergency department from the mental health client's perspective. *International Journal of Mental Health Nursing* 16, 126–131.

Clarke, D. E., Hughes, L., Browne, A. M., & Motluk, L. (2005). Psychiatric emergency nurses in the emergency department: The success of the Winnipeg, Canada, experience. *Journal of Emergency Nursing* 31 (4), 351–356.

Clinton, M., & Hazelton, M. (2000). Scoping the prospects of Australian mental health nursing final article, in a series of four. *Australian and New Zealand Journal of Mental Health Nursing* 9 (4), 159–165.

DeSanto-Madeya, S. (2007). Using case studies based on a nursing conceptual model to teach medical-surgical nursing. *Nursing Science Quarterly* 20 (4), 324–329.

Dunphy, L. M., Youngkin, E. Q., & Smith, N. K. (2004). Advanced Practice Nursing: Doing what had to be done. In L. A. Joel (ed.), *Advanced Practice Nursing: Essentials for Role Development.* F.A. Davis Company: Philadelphia.

Eales, S., Callahan, P., & Johnson, B. (2006). Service users and other stakeholders' evaluation of a liaison mental health service in an accident and emergency department and a general hospital setting. *Journal of Psychiatric and Mental Health Nursing* 13, 70–71.

Elsom, S., Happell, B., & Manias, E. (2005). Mental health nurse practitioner: Expanded or advanced? *International Journal of Mental Health Nursing* 14, 181–186.

Ferraz, H., & Wellman, N. (2008). The integration of solution focused brief therapy principles in nursing; a literature review. *Journal of Psychiatric and Mental Health Nursing* 15, 37–54.

Fisher, J. (2005). Mental health nurse practitioners in Australia: Improving access to quality mental health care. *International Journal of Mental Health Nursing* 14, 222–229.

Gardner, G., Dunn, S., Carryer, J., & Gardner, A. (2006). Competency and capability: Imperative for nurse practitioner education. *Australian Journal of Advanced Nursing* 24 (1), 8–14.

Gardner, A., & Gardner, G. (2005). A trial of nurse practitioner scope of practice. *Journal of Advanced Nursing* 49 (2), 135–145.

Gardner, G., & Gardner, A. (2007). Living with chronic illness. In M. McAllister (ed.) *Solution Focused Nursing: Rethinking Practice.* Palgrave: Hampshire, UK, pp. 143–153.

Gillette, J., Bucknell, M., & Meegan, E. (1996). *Evaluation of Psychiatric Nurse Consultancy in Emergency Departments Project.* RMIT Faculty of Nursing, Melbourne.

Happell, B., & Platania-Phung, C. (2005). Mental health issues within the general health care system: Implications for the nursing profession. *Australian Journal of Advanced Nursing* 22 (3), 41–47.

Henderson, A. (2007). Expanding nurses' capabilities in acute care. In M. McAllister (ed.) *Solution Focused Nursing: Rethinking Practice.* Palgrave: Hampshire, UK, pp. 103–115.

Heslop, L., Elsom, S., & Parker, N. (2000). Improving continuity of care across psychiatric and emergency services: Combining patient data within a participatory action research framework. *Journal of Advanced Nursing* 31 (1), 135–143.

Hosnay, Z., Wellerman, N., & Lowe, T. (2007). Fostering a culture of engagement: A pilot study of the outcomes of training mental health nurses working in two UK admission units in brief solution-focused therapy techniques. *Journal of Psychiatric and Mental Health Nursing* 14, 688–695.

Hughes, L. G., & Clarke, D. E. (2002). Psychiatric nurses in hospital emergency departments. *The Canadian Nurse* 98 (10), 23–26.

Kerrison, S. A., & Chapman, R. (2007). What general emergency nurses want to know about mental health patients presenting to their emergency department. *Accident and Emergency Nursing* 15 (1), 48–55.

Lamprecht, H., Laydon, C., McQuillin, C., Wiseman, S., Williams, L., Gash, A., & Reilly, J. (2007). Single-session solution-focused brief therapy and self-harm. *Journal of Psychiatric and Mental Health Nursing* 14, 601–602.

McDonough, S., Wynaden, D., Finn, M., McGowan, S., Chapman, R., & Hood, S. (2004). Emergency department mental health triage consultancy service: An evaluation of the first year of the service. *Accident and Emergency Nursing* 12, 31–38.

Middleton, S., Allnutt, J., Griffiths, R., McMaster, R., O'Connell, J., & Hillege, S. (2007). Identifying measures for evaluating new models of nursing care: A survey of NSW nurse practitioners. *International Journal of Nursing Practice* 13, 331–340.

Musker, M. (2007). Learning difficulties and solution focused nursing. In M. McAllister (ed.) *Solution Focused Nursing: Rethinking Practice.* Palgrave: Hampshire, UK, pp. 77–87.

Macdonald, A. (2007). *Solution-Focused Therapy. Theory, Research & Practice.* Sage: Los Angeles.

McAllister, M. (2003). Doing practice differently: Solution-focused nursing. *Journal of Advanced Nursing* 41 (6), 528–535.

McAllister, M. (2007). Youth work. In M. McAllister (ed.) *Solution Focused Nursing: Rethinking Practice.* Palgrave: Hampshire, UK, pp. 88–102.

McAllister, M., Zimmer-Gembeck, M., Moyle, W., & Billett, S. (2008). Working effectively with clients who self-injure using a solution focused approach. *International Emergency Nursing* 16, 272–279.

Pearson, A., & Peels, S. (2002). The nurse practitioner. *International Journal of Nursing Practice* 8, S5–S10.

Roberts, D. (1997). Liaison mental health nursing: Origins, definition and prospects. *Journal of Advanced Nursing* 25 (1), 101–108.

Roberts, D. (2002). Working models for practice. In S. Regal, & D. Roberts (eds.) *Mental Health Liaison; A Handbook for Nurses and Health Professionals.* Bailliere: Tindall, Edinburgh, pp. 23–42.

Rowe, J., & Barnes, M. (2007). Families in transition: Early parenting. In M. McAllister (ed.) *Solution Focused Nursing: Rethinking Practice.* Palgrave: Hampshire, UK, pp. 49–62.

Sinclair, L., Hunter, R., Hagen, S., Nelson, D., & Hunt, J. (2006). How effective are mental health nurses in A & E departments? *Emergency Medical Journal* 23, 687–692.

Stevenson, C., Jackson, S., & Barker, P. (2003). Finding solutions through empowerment: A preliminary study of a solution orientated approach to nursing in acute psychiatric settings. *Journal of Psychiatric and Mental Health Nursing* 10, 688–696.

Torn, A., & McNichol, E. (1996). Can a mental health nurse be a nurse practitioner? *Nursing Standard* 11 (2), 39–42.

Walsh, K., & Moss, C. (2007). Solution focused mental health nursing. In M. McAllister (ed.) *Solution Focused Nursing.* Palgrave: Hampshire, UK, pp. 116–126.

Walsh, K., Moss, C., Lawless, J., Mckelvie, R., & Duncan, L. (2008). Puzzling practice: A strategy for working with clinical practice issues. *International Journal of Nursing Practice* 14, 94–100.

Wand, T. (2004). Mental health liaison nurses in the emergency department: On-site expertise and enhanced coordination of care. *Australian Journal of Advanced Nursing* 22 (2), 25–31.

Wand, T., & Fisher, J. (2006). The mental health nurse practitioner in the emergency department: An Australian experience. *International Journal of Mental Health Nursing* 15 (3), 201–208.

Wand, T., & Happell, B. (2001). The mental health nurse: Contributing to improved outcomes for patients in the emergency department. *Accident and Emergency Nursing* 9, 1–11.

Wand, T., & Schaecken, P. (2006). Consumer evaluation of a mental health liaison nurse service. *Contemporary Nurse* 21 (1), 14–21.

Wand, T., & White, K. (2007a). Progression of the mental health nurse practitioner role in Australia. *Journal of Psychiatric and Mental Health Nursing* 14 (7), 644–651.

Wand, T., & White, K. (2007b). Examining models of mental health service delivery in the emergency department. *Australian and New Zealand Journal of Psychiatry* 41 (10), 784–791.

Wortans, J., Happell, B., & Johnstone, H. (2006). The role of the nurse practitioner in psychiatric/mental health nursing: Exploring consumer satisfaction. *Journal of Psychiatric & Mental Health Nursing* 13 (1), 78–84.

Chapter 5

Developing simulated scenarios with simulated patients to enhance the acquisition of therapeutic helping skills

Sam Samociuk and Anne Lawton

■ Introduction

This chapter will explore the use of simulated patients (SPs) to create an 'as if in practice' learning scenario to stimulate students into using basic therapeutic helping skills. Two therapeutic approaches provide the framework for developing these skills: the person-centred and psychodynamic approaches (also see Chapter 6 for other elements of the psychodynamic approach). The students we are referring to in this chapter are mental health nursing students, who at the start of the second year of their three-year course are introduced to SP work and are encouraged to use a person-centred approach, and at third year have a second opportunity to work with SPs using a psychodynamic approach.

The chapter will offer a rationale for utilising SPs in helping scenarios, an outline of the processes of preparation for all parties and a discussion of the issues arising. Throughout the chapter we offer dialogue on our specific experiences relating to the points we raise.

■ Background

The training of health and social care professionals in communication and basic helping skills has become an increasingly vital component of education programmes for a range of professionals (GMC, 2002). The emergence

68

of the client-centred approach in the 1940s and 1950s saw the movement towards acquiring knowledge and skills through a direct and experiential focus (Rogers, 1959). The challenge of developing courses which promoted the acquisition of skills in the classroom prior to the reality of supervised practice was and still is evident. For example, in the 1990s counselling skills were taught as a combination of verbal and non-verbal responses, often taking the form of micro-skills training (Dryden, 1991; Inskipp, 1996). The experiential agenda required the students, through structured classroom activities and role-play scenarios, to explore and engage in a method of learning which embraced not only the cognitive and psychomotor domains but also the affective domain.

An essential component of all education for health care professionals is the belief that in order to understand others it is first important to understand and reflect upon 'self' (Dryden and Thorne, 1991). However, self-awareness is not always directly addressed but undoubtedly students are affected at a personal level by their experiences in these experiential situations. Whether or not this is sufficient to allow students to develop as responsive, empathic professionals is unclear. Hanna and Fins (2006) argue that the depth of interpersonal relating is achieved only when students are exposed to the diversity, tragedy and joy of real people:

> I recall one student whose struggle was almost palpable. She was a student who had several years of experience as a support worker and had survived several traumatic life events. She had rightly developed a confidence and self-vision as someone who was competent and skilled at communicating with people and indeed this was true. She was adept at building relationships with people particularly at a social and supportive level. However, her ability to transfer her skills to a more formal, although simulated, therapeutic setting provided an unexpected challenge. Having faith in her skills, she now found herself having to display and receive comments regarding these skills and at times this feedback was not affirming but (constructively) critical and challenging. As these sessions progressed she journeyed through uncertainty, what do I say? What should I pick up on? Can't we just have a chat?; got stuck at several cross roads, past, present, empathy, sympathy, counter-transference, here and now; and sometimes found herself immersed in human emotion, both her own and others' but eventually she emerged with a new sense of her skills and capabilities which added to her existing formulation of self rather than undermining or deskilling her.

The counselling model of skills training usually entails the students identifying themselves as both client and counsellor. Alternating between these roles, the student can either work on their own material or role-play a client. Dryden (1991) outlines the difficulties of using this type of personalised training caused by the insertion of a relationship dynamic which does not reflect real practice. However, using this method of skills training can provide students with a sense of the vulnerability experienced by many people seeking help as it engages the student in a real 'here and now' encounter. This may be the only opportunity students have of experiencing their own responses and reactions to being the client. It is therefore a challenge to educators across professions to find ways of ensuring personal development is attended to.

■ The use of simulation

Simulated patients have been used in medical education for numerous years as a strategy to ensure that health and social care students are prepared for the skilled work of their profession (Kilminster et al., 2005). Collins and Harden (2004) identify an SP as a person who is carefully coached to present the symptoms and signs of an actual patient thus providing what Adamo (2003) refers to as realistic and three-dimensional portrayals of actual patients. The use of SP makes session facilitation a much freer experience, with the lecturers able to concentrate fully on the student's interactions and managing the overall process. Students are able to relate to the SP as a 'real' client at least in the sense of a first encounter with someone they had not met before.

■ Funding and recruitment of SPs

Fortunately, in our University, the Strategic Health Authority supported the use of SPs and had gone through a tendering process to establish a provider for the SPs in our region; this was a local theatre company who mainly provided actors. These individuals came from a variety of occupational backgrounds (teaching, social work, medicine, counselling and full-time acting) and had a range of acting experience which included stage work, educational performances and appearances on television. All had experience of being an SP in health and social care educational settings, and some had experience of either using services or being a carer or any combination of these.

In the initial stages the theatre company was contracted to provide 4,000 hours of SP work across the region. This arrangement continued for some time but was eventually changed and funding from the Strategic Health Authority (SHA) withdrawn; this then placed the burden of funding directly on each university department if they wished this work to continue. In fact it was only when the cost became apparent to those championing this work that the true extent of the financial implications became a real and significant issue.

■ Preparation of actors

Many of the SPs are experienced in working with medical students as simulators or standardised patients in various assessments and clinical examinations. However, the use of SPs explored in this chapter is novel. The focus for the SPs was on the students' skill development rather than on assessment. To achieve this they were asked to play the same patient for a number of sessions spread over a series of weeks, rather than the more contained simulations they were used to, which may involve repetition of a simulated encounter several times in one session.

The SP roles were written by the lecturers who had clinical practice roles; this went someway to ensuring the validity and authenticity of the roles. The company took the responsibility of allocating appropriately experienced SPs for this work and the SPs were briefed beforehand by the lecturing staff. It was clear from the SPs' feedback that they found this work both exciting and challenging, and the need to spend time to debrief the SPs was particularly evident in the third module. During this module the SPs were required to adopt the role of someone who had or was experiencing a particularly distressing time in their life; for example, recently being given a diagnosis of incurable cancer, having experienced physical violence or recently being bereaved. Debriefing is particularly pertinent to this type of role as the vulnerability of the SP to the emotional impact of the work has previously been documented (Hardoff and Schonmann, 2001).

The strength of using SPs is that it allows students to work with individuals who are not known to them and who, at their best, convincingly role-play a character that is believable and authentic. Although it is not intended to replace practice, the experience mirrors that of practice whilst also providing an arena for students to practice skills without the fear of offending their colleagues or of saying the 'wrong thing' to someone who is presenting with real problems.

■ Preparation of students

There is a need to prepare the students for two aspects of this work: one is the acquisition of basic therapeutic helping skills; the second is preparing the students for the simulated encounter. In the example explored here, mental health nursing students drew on Heron's *Six Category Intervention Analysis* (Heron, 1990), utilising the catalytic category of interventions, which include the use of open and closed questioning, reflection, summarizing, paraphrasing, self-disclosure and empathic responding.

Mental health work is by its very nature concerned with the affective domain of human experience. However, learning how to be with someone in distress is part of the emotional labour of all health and social care work (McQueen, 2004; Freshwater and Stickley, 2004) requiring that students of those professions not be afraid of asking sensitive questions and be able to identify the cues that are given by the patient/simulator. In the early stages of this work the students tend to be more focused on the 'factual content' of people's stories, and whilst familiar with asking questions to elicit information from patients, they are less skilled at communicating their understanding empathically and paying attention to the emotional content of someone's story.

These sessions also help the learning group to develop; to this end ice-breaker and group development exercises are undertaken, with some of these videotaped and replayed to the group as a means of defusing their anxieties and helping them to become familiar with this medium. The second aspect of preparation is outlining for the students the format and structure of the simulated sessions.

■ Format of the SP sessions

Students undertaking this module are of a varied demographic; age, sex, ethnic background and level of experience in mental health care are all variable factors. The majority of students would not have not participated in similar training activities and one may argue that without exception they are in the position of novice. The student group is divided into three or four smaller groups for the simulated sessions, and remain in these groups throughout the module.

During the first module that uses SPs the context is a first meeting with a new referral to a primary care or community-based mental health nurse, and a person-centred approach is used. Each group has an SP to interview using a 'serial counselling' training technique. This requires each student to carry out a five-minute portion of the interview. After five minutes, the interview stops and the feedback process begins, providing an opportunity for the group to consider what the next interviewer might address. The next student then continues the interview and after five minutes the same process ensues. Each student's input is videotaped on his or her own tape so that they may review their tape, compare their perceptions with the feedback received and use this to complete their overall review, which is presented to the group later in the module.

■ Facilitator observations

Students come to this work with mixed abilities; these observations are an attempt to capture some of the struggles students have in developing a more 'person-centred' approach to their interventions.

One student attended the module preparation sessions and so was present when we outlined and discussed the need to connect with the client by listening, exploring and acknowledging the client's story through the use of Heron's catalytic skills of questioning, reflection, summarising, paraphrasing and empathy.

Buchanan-Barker and Barker (2005) refer to the need for 'bridging' with the client; initially described as engagement but further developed to articulate, through metaphor, the art of making a connection between the nurse/therapist and the person who is in a difficult–to-reach emotional landscape (see chapter 3).

> This student gathered information from the client and started to lay the foundations for her bridge to take shape, however, very quickly for each forward step, she incrementally began to lay more and more explosive devices, unwittingly designed to destroy not only the bridge, but the landmass where the potential for foundations needed to be solid.

Many students seem to believe that they need to become problem solvers and solution givers for all situations; this is a basic bridge design fault which metaphorically has two designers/builders, each starting at their respective ends of the project and each with a different plan, one for a swing bridge and the other for a cantilever construction. Coupled with this basic design fault, it only took a very short time for the devices to start exploding. The detonators for these came in the form of interventions which did not acknowledge the client's predicaments or emotional state.

> You have a supportive family, a good job and a loving husband – you will soon be okay, there is no need to feel depressed.

This is the reassurance of the unconfident builder, who on hearing the concerns of the client still pursues *their* own plan whilst not paying attention to the client's concerns. Another detonator, frequently activated, is the referral to another service. There is no doubt that in mental health care a range of disciplines and services exist to offer specific help for a person's needs and these should be used appropriately, with health professionals knowing their limitations and referring on to others. However, if early in the therapeutic encounter the builder says, 'I know another builder who can do this for you, I will send you to them', the possibility of connecting with the client is dashed because there has not been time for the client to develop trust in the builder's judgement and therefore is likely to feel abandoned and less likely to trust the next builder who approaches. The new builder needs to temper their anxiety with patience and keep their focus on the needs of the client; this may involve repeated renegotiation of their needs, changes to their plans and occasional disagreement. But this process should give the basis for a functional bridge which connects the two parties; the focus then can change to the flow of 'traffic' between both sides and the quality of the journey. Many of the students successfully achieved the match between planning and bridge building; some already had good bridging skills while others had to develop these, but most improved on these skills over a relatively short period of time.

The recent inclusion of an Objective Structured Clinical Examination (OSCE) that involves a re-enactment of these sessions – apart from it being done on an individual basis with each student having three ten-minute slots equating to the beginning, middle and end of a counselling session – has gone some way to reinforce the importance of such skill development within the world of academia and the high priority given to theoretical knowledge. However, the inclusion of an OSCE as a means of testing the acquisition of specific core helping skills potentially shifts the focus towards an emphasis on specific skills, rather than the therapeutic process and the natural emergence of the qualities associated with this approach.

■ Feedback process

Students engage in exercises to help them understand the principles of feedback; the model used is based on Hawkins and Shohet's acronym CORBS, which stands for *Clear, Owned, Regular, Balanced and Specific* (Hawkins and Shohet, 2000). Within the simulations the format for feedback is that the student gives their view of their performance, what worked well and what did not, the SP, in role, gives their reaction to the interaction, and finally the group members and the facilitator are invited to give feedback to the student. Likewise, the student's peer group are encouraged to give written feedback based on their observation using a structured checklist based on the catalytic category (Heron, 1990) and Egan's SOLER format (Egan, 1998).

■ Video work

There is a good argument for using video to capture skills training sessions as this provides the student with a tangible record of their work. This may then be used for reflection on their skills development and as a personal archive which may be useful when providing evidence for accreditation of prior learning (APL). However, the mere mention of video does tend to raise participants' anxieties! Students are assured that the video is there as their personal tool for reflection as it is not seen by anyone else and it is their decision whether to keep it or delete it once the sessions have finished.

Students usually show progress in developing their therapeutic skills and approach over the course of the simulated sessions. However, some have struggled with the shift from data collection and problem-solving to creating the 'necessary and sufficient conditions' (Rogers, 1959) for personal exploration whilst demonstrating understanding and empathy for the patient.

■ Student feedback

The SP work is completed by the mid-point of the module and evaluated using two questionnaires, one related to the SP and the processes of the work and another more generally to the module. The students' comments and ratings seem to confirm what O'Connor et al. (1999) found in their study, namely that their learning was enhanced by the actual experience of working with a simulator they did not know and that the feedback from them and the lecturing staff was extremely valuable. For some students this revalidated for them what mental health nursing was primarily concerned with. The students also commented that their high anxiety at the beginning reduced as they became more familiar with the process and confident that they were in a safe environment, the small groups being a key component of that safety. As a brief flavour of the feedback the evaluations from students from a recent cohort are considered:

> (I was) apprehensive at first. Didn't really think that I would get much out of the experience as the setting was not real. However, I did find the whole experience beneficial and (it) gave me the opportunity to put skills into practice and receive feedback.

Another student

> Found it a valuable experience and learnt much from it.

One student commented on how

> "Tense and nerve wracking" it was.

They also reported that it boosted their self-confidence.
 Three students specifically identified the use of video as being important to their learning. One wrote,

> I was definitely able to develop skills and reflect back using the video.

The approach and methods of teaching utilising SPs is transferable to any number of different educational settings and clinical contexts. One way of extending the authenticity of this work and grounding it in the specific professional context would be to have staff and service users jointly writing SP outlines and scenarios to closely replicate the types of practice the students would encounter.

■ Psychodynamic approach

Students progress through the course with exposure to different psychological approaches; at the end of the second year the students undertake a module which uses the psychodynamic perspective as the underpinning knowledge framework for the simulated sessions. McLeod (2003) argues that the psychodynamic perspective is often resistive to the notion of skill development preferring to place the focus upon the emerging relationship between therapist and client and the complex and unconscious dynamics of that relationship. McLeod (2003) suggests that practitioners need to be equipped with a theoretical perspective through which to understand their work with clients. It is this focus that is addressed during this module. It is intended that the experience will maintain and enhance the acquisition of the core helping skills (Heron, 1990) whilst offering a perspective that enables reflection and understanding and possible intervention from an alternative viewpoint.

Much has been written about the integration of theories and approaches which create new and distinctive models of therapeutic helping. O'Leary and Murphy (2006) endorse the case for integration and clearly identify this area as a distinct discipline. It is not intended that students embark on such a complicated journey at this stage but rather that they are exposed to a theoretical perspective which develops their understanding and ability to respond to people with complex needs. One of the most useful aspects of this process of integration is the students' increasing understanding of their own counter-transference reactions, which helps them to increase their empathy and understanding of service users.

> I have over the years encountered many students who have commented upon how helpless or frustrated they feel when listening to their client's story. On examination they have been able to recognise that perhaps they are internalising the client's feelings of helplessness and frustration. Undoubtedly there have been times when students have felt very emotional in response to the client's story and again have been able to understand that possibly they are feeling the client's distress. This alternative perspective seems to offer a way forward for the students as they show a greater level of understanding of both their own responses and those of the client.

The intention is not to prepare people to be therapists but to highlight the potential importance of past life events for current functioning and to recognise that some behaviour may be an outward reflection of unconscious conflicts. Klamen and Yudkowsky (2002) identify this area as a core feature in developing the use of SPs in an Introduction to Psychotherapy course. It is also a way of encouraging students to view human motivation in a more constructive way, as a potential means of communicating distress, rather than dismissing behaviour as 'attention seeking' or 'manipulative' (Hamilton and Manias, 2006). Thus the introduction of psychodynamic concepts provides a framework for understanding the potentially complex presentations of individuals which can often be mystifying and challenging for practitioners. This is reflected in the student's clinical experience at the time of undertaking the module. They are actively engaged with working with people with more complex problems in their clinical practice.

■ Preparation of the actors

The SP is given a character outline with details of past life events and current problems. Coaching of the SP by the module team occurs as the relationship between the students and the SP develops. The SP is encouraged to offer reactions and responses which highlight defence mechanisms or relationship issues which reflect past life experiences. Further direction is given to the SP if necessary; for example, the SP may be asked to release specific personal or family information (as part of their role) to enable the students to identify psychodynamic themes. As well as the coaching and support offered to the SP, there is still considerable latitude for the SP to interpret the internal experiences of the character from their own frame of reference.

SPs often comment upon the challenge of maintaining the character over seven weeks. As a consequence of the often unpredictable process the lecturers are presented with what Wakefield et al. (2003) describe as an immediate learning tool. The actor brings a degree of spontaneity which challenges both lecturers and students to unpick possible dynamics and reflect them back to the SP. Spontaneity in the simulated sessions means that actors are using their personality, background, life experiences and expectations of the students to inform their interpretation of the character; if channelled to the needs of the students this can bring to life the character. In some circumstances the SP becomes immersed in their interpretation and is no longer able to adapt to the requirements of the sessions. At times it seems there is almost a power struggle between the facilitator and actor as to the best way to convey the various dimensions of the role. In some ways this mirrors the therapeutic process where the expectations of helper and client are not always mutual and clearly understood from both perspectives. It is important to maintain a clear dialogue with the SP and to openly address any difficulties so that they do not interfere with the simulated encounter. This, however, can be easier said than done.

On one occasion I worked with a very experienced and skilled actor who clearly had ideas about the role and the way to play the role. Unfortunately, this did not always match with my expectations. No matter how many times we discussed the session beforehand and highlighted areas to emphasise or directions to take, the actor just went his own way. Frustrations mounted and it began to feel like the actor who would not take direction and the director who would not allow the actor spontaneity to develop the character. Dialogue continued but to little effect. The students continued apparently unaware of these power dynamics but at an unconscious level I suspect that these frustrations leaked out and will have impacted upon their responses. This is an aspect of working with simulated patients that I had not anticipated, the complexities of working in this way continue to unfold and surprise and must be attended to by some form of reflective structure, debriefing sessions or regular clinical supervision.

■ Preparation of students

The students self-select into two small groups and are expected to have 10 minutes each to work with the client followed by feedback from their peers and tutors. A minimum of five students are expected to work with the client in any given session, mirroring the 50-minute hour of counselling and psychotherapy. The SP is asked to give feedback in terms of a personal reflection of how they are feeling in the here and now. There is an expectation that the students will be able to engage and utilise appropriate therapeutic helping skills which they will be able to use within the 10 minutes allocated. They are encouraged to develop their ability to reflect upon the dynamics of the relationship, and start to acquire the quality of being what Casement (1990) refers to as an 'internal supervisor'. This enables the students to focus upon their emotional responses to the character and move to the paradoxical position of intimacy yet distance from the person (Casement, 1990).

Integrated into the module are two theory sessions where psychodynamic principles are discussed and applied to the work done with the SP. Some of the theorists referred are Milan (1995), Casement (1990), Bowlby (1993) and Winnicott (1957, 1965). The intention is to provide the students with an insight into this approach in a way that makes the theory accessible. Small case studies and self-reflective exercises are used to stimulate the student's interest and motivation. Attention is paid particularly to defence mechanisms, transference and counter-transference, and therapeutic boundaries. At the end of the module students are expected to write a 3000-word essay on one of these areas and apply the principles either to their work with the SP or to a client from clinical practice. Individual sessions are also offered to support students with this.

Students are expected to use a videotape so they have a record of their work which they are able to reflect upon at a later date. Emphasising the importance of past experiences can sometimes trigger personal responses from students which are responded to sensitively. This may mean spending individual time with the student or even referring them to other student support services. Discussion of the process often raises the students' anxiety with comments such as 'I'll never be able to do ten minutes', 'I can't do it with everyone watching.' Interestingly, the focus of the anxiety is generally upon performing in front of peers rather than being videoed.

■ Student group

Despite some anxieties most students comment upon the usefulness of this way of learning and are willing to get involved. It is important for the facilitator to hear these anxieties but to offer containment to them mirroring the approach. Students are still expected to attend and to participate. If they 'get stuck' during their ten minutes they are able to freeze the session and ask for help from colleagues. Some students do use this mechanism and are usually able to continue after a brief pause.

As this module occurs at the end of the second year the constituent members are usually set and the group has by then progressed through its own developmental stages. However, Tuckman and Jensen (1977) argue that as groups move through their phases in their own way and time, so the lecturers cannot assume that the group is at a point of performing or has moved beyond the storming stage. The introduction of this structure may in itself challenge the norms already set by the group and precipitate the emergence of hidden or new dynamics. Issues of inclusion and exclusion sometimes develop. The structure of the serial counselling does place huge expectations upon the student to 'expose' their skills in front of their tutor and peers. This here-and-now experience seems to compliment the learning process and indirectly allows the student to reflect upon self and their inner experiences of participation in the process.

■ Feedback issues

One of the main advantages of using SPs is the instant feedback they are able to provide. Wakefield et al. (2003) emphasise the value students place on this aspect of learning. Dacre et al. (2004) go as far as to argue that feedback is the essential ingredient of communication skills courses and is more effective than observing experts or videotapes or discussing issues. Students receive feedback from their peer group, lecturers and the SP, which is immediate to and focused on the students' interactions. As Inskipp (1996) argues, providing constructive and skilled feedback is an essential aspect of helping within a professional context; to be helpful, feedback needs to be supportive and constructive. Students are often over-enthusiastic about their colleagues' interactions or say very little so the student is left not knowing how they came across or which areas they need to develop. There can be an over-reliance upon the tutor's feedback, students feeling judged if their remarks do not tally with those of the tutor. Klamen and Yudkowsky (2002) suggest that positive aspects of interactions should be highlighted first so that students feel supported when working experientially. Interestingly, it is often the positive comments that are most difficult for students to accept.

> I recall one student offering an excellent 10-minute interaction with the SP, utilising a range of appropriate skills which were insightful and empathic. These were clearly recognised and fed back to her by all concerned. On receipt of this feedback her only comment was, 'O.K but what did I do wrong?' This was disappointing at two levels: she struggled to acknowledge her skills and qualities; she had also internalised a view of right or wrong rather than a more fluid interpretation of trying to understand 'what do I uniquely bring to the relationship' and 'how might I understand and refine this?'

Feedback from the SP is very valuable and immediate. This has often been most effective when it was spontaneous and seemed to come from the SP's real projection to being a service user. Comments about appropriateness of dress have had particular impact. One SP, in role, challenged a student dressed in torn jeans and wearing a baseball cap:

> What are you doing dressed like that? Do you think that makes me feel as though I can trust you? I can't even see you properly.

The student did not attend the session in torn jeans and a baseball cap again. Clearly the student seemed to respond to this direct feedback; however, whether this is a representation of the real relationship or the transference/counter-transference relationship is open to debate.

■ Limitations

Although the use of SPs has many advantages it is important to acknowledge potential drawbacks. Hanna and Fins (2006) argue firmly that the use of SPs in medical training fosters the emergence of the simulated 'doctor'. They suggest that medical students learn to perform rather than to genuinely engage with people in a helping relationship. However, as Hanna and Fins (2006) propose, it is the real-life encounters where most learning emerges. The authenticity of the character is vital for engaging students in this process. The more believable the character the more able the students are to develop rapport and feel involved with the client (Klamen and Yudkowsky, 2002). If the actors are able to emotionally experience the character and display this then the students become increasingly engaged with the SP and forget the 'unreal' aspect of the situation. Difficulties have arisen when the personality or presentation of the SP has not been congruent with the character they are portraying.

When this has occurred it has been difficult for students to differentiate between the character and the person and therefore to be clear who they are responding to. The dynamics of the student–actor relationship may produce real transference issues, or stimulate real issues for the actor, which result in avoidance or defensive strategies which are beyond the remit of the students. As facilitators, there is a need to optimise learning whilst maintaining the well-being of the actor. The theory sessions have provided an outlet for discussion of this type of dilemma. Klamen and Yudkowsky (2002), in their use of SPs in psychotherapy training, encourage SPs to develop their own role or use personal experience for the encounter. They report that most of the SPs used their own personal material. This would seem to negate some of the difficulties identified and offer a valuable alternative for this particular approach. Similarly, the actors' expectations of students vary and so it is again important to brief SPs particularly on how to respond if the students are struggling. Again it is a balance between responding in a way that facilitates learning without deskilling students to the extent that they become paralysed and unable to respond.

Facilitator and actor fatigue is also a potential issue which can affect the process of the sessions. If the same characters are used there is a tendency to become over-familiar with the issues of that character and to respond automatically, rather than truly listening to the story each time it is presented. Although it is useful for the actors to develop their roles it can lose impact on the fourth or fifth time of listening to that character. Eagles et al. (2007) support this view suggesting that once a script or performance has been perfected it is tempting not to change it so that teaching sessions may become outdated or repetitive.

Undoubtedly, involvement in this module is potentially emotionally exhausting for the actors involved (Eagles et al., 2007). Their role is maintained over seven sessions so the character is well developed from both a complex mental health perspective and often a traumatic past history. At times actors may identify with the role or the character's experiences. The actors often tell us that they rely on their own life situations to help them add depth to the character. This level of involvement is admirable but could leave individuals vulnerable to emotional turmoil and even distress. Therefore, it is important to debrief after each session and provide time for SPs to address any issues they may have. It is often useful for the actors and facilitators to share interpretations and reactions to the session. As the psychodynamic approach particularly places emphasis on the emerging relationship between therapist and client, it could be argued that the use of SPs can produce a stilted, mechanistic view of therapeutic helping. There seems to be an inherent danger that the student's own personality could be stifled by the emphasis on skills and theories. The spontaneity of the student and their ability to respond as an individual may be compromised by the constraining focus on skills and the tension of the situation. However, this is balanced by the attention paid to both individual and collective discussion and reflection upon the experience.

■ Conclusion

The development of therapeutic helping skills for any professional requires patience, diligence and commitment. There is little doubt that when student practitioners become evermore exposed to simulated situations which are safe and structured this facilitates authentic experiential learning. There is also a real opportunity for the students to begin their journey of self development, which will give them an increasing awareness of their abilities and the meaning of true engagement with clients.

References

Adamo, G. (2003) Simulated and standardized patients in OSCEs: Achievements and challenges 1992–2003. *Medical Teacher*, 25(3), 262–270, Taylor & Francis Health Sciences.

Bowlby, J. (1993) *A Secure Base: Clinical Applications of Attachment Theory*. Routledge: London.

Buchanan-Barker, P. and Barker, P. (2005) Observation: The original sin of mental health nursing? *Journal of Psychiatric and MH nursing*, 12, 541–549.

Casement, P. (1990) *On Learning from the Patient*. Routledge: London.

Collins, J.P. and Harden, P.M. (2004) The use of real patients, simulated patients and simulators in clinical examinations. AMEE Medical Education Guide No. 13.

Dacre, J., Richardson, J., Noble, L., Stephens, K. and Parker, N. (2004) Communication skills training in postgraduate medicine; the development of a new course. *Postgraduate Medical Journal*, 80, 711–715.

Dryden, W. (1991) *Training and Supervision* vol. 3. Whurr Pubilsher: London.

Department of Health (1997) National Service Framework for Mental Health.

Dryden, W. and Thorne, B. (1991) *Training and Supervision for Counselling in Action*. Sage: London.

Eagles, J.M., Calder, S.A., Wilson, S., Murdoch, J.M. and Sclare, P.D. (2007) Simulated patients in undergraduate education in psychiatry. *Psychiatric Bulletin*, 31, 187–190.

Egan, G. (1998) *The Skilled Helper*. (6th Edn.) Brooks: Cole, London.

Freshwater, D. and Stickley, T. (2004) The heart of the art: Emotional intelligence in nurse education. *Nursing Inquiry*, 11, 91–98, Blackwell Publishing Ltd.

General Medical Council (2002) *Tomorrow's Doctors*. GMC: London.

Hardoff, D. and Schonmann, S. (2001) Training physicians in communication skills with adolescents using teenage actors as simulated patients. *Medical Education*, 35, 206–210, Blackwell Science Ltd.

Hamilton, B. and Manias, E. (2006) 'She's manipulative and he's right off': A critical analysis of psychiatric nurses' oral and written language in the acute inpatient setting. *International Journal of Mental Health Nursing*, 15, 84–92.

Hanna, M. and Fins, J. (2006) Power and communication: Why simulation teaching ought to be complemented by experiential and humanistic learning (Viewpoint) *Academic Medicine*, 81(3), 265–270.

Heron, J. (1990) *Helping the Client*. Sage: London.

Inskipp, F. (1996) *Skills Training for Counselling*. Cassell: London.

Kilminster, S., Morris, P., Simpson, E., Thistlethwaite, J. and Ewart, B. (2005) Using patients' experiences in medical education: First steps in inter-professional training? In McAndrew, S. and Warne, T. (eds) *Using Patient Experience in Nurse Education*. Palgrave Macmillan: Hampshire, England.

Klamen, D.L. and Yudkowsky, R. (2002) Using Standardized Patients for Formative Feedback in an Introduction to Psychotherapy Course. *Academic Psychiatry*, 26(3), 168–172.

McLeod, J. (2003) *An Introduction to Counselling Skills*. (3rd Edn.) Open University Press: Berkshire.

McQueen, A.C.H. (2004) Emotional intelligence in nursing work. *Journal of Advanced Nursing*, 47(1), 101–108, Blackwell Publishing Ltd.

Milan, H.D. (1995) *Individual Psychotherapy and the Science of Psychodynamics*. Butterworth-Heinemann: Oxford.

O'Connor, F.W., Albert, M.L. and Thomas, M.D. (1999) Incorporating standardized patients into a psychosocial nurse practitioner programme. *Archive Psychiatric Nursing*, 13(5), 240–247.

O'Leary, E. and Murphy, M. (eds) (2006) *New Approaches to Integration in Psychotherapy*. Routledge: London.

Rogers, C. (1959) *Client Centred Therapy*. Prentice Hall: New York.

Tuckman, B.W. and Jensen, M.A.C. (1977) Stages of small group development revisited. *Group and Organisational Studies*, 2, 419–427.

Wakefield, A., Cooke, S. and Boggis, C. (2003) Learning together: Use of simulated patients with nursing and medical students for breaking bad news. *International Journal of Palliative Nursing*, 9(1), 32–38.

Winnicott, D. (1957) *Primary Maternal Preoccupation in Collected Papers: Through Paediatrics to Psychoanalysis*. Tavistock: London.

Winnicott, D. (1965) *The Maturational Process and the Facilitating Environment*. Hogarth: London, pp. 140–152.

Chapter 6

Knowing me and understanding you through discourse

Marie Crowe

■ Introduction

This chapter will explore how health and social care workers can work with people in distress to develop a therapeutic alliance that takes into account the sociocultural context of the alliance. Distress may be caused by mental, emotional and physical illness and social problems in the here and now. However, distress may be experienced in the here and now as a reminiscence of previous traumatic experience. This chapter explores the principles of psychodynamic and discursive approaches to knowing me and understanding you through the development of the 'therapeutic' alliance. Specific emphasis will be given to how such principles can be applied to a case example in such a way that best enables the student to translate them into their developing practice. Throughout the discussion on the case example reflective questions are posed for students to consider how discourses have influenced their own sense of self and their practice.

Specifically this chapter will explore a discursive approach to the therapeutic alliance. This approach can be described as a process involving meanings and how they are expressed. The therapeutic alliance involves mutual constructions of new meanings and subject positions through dialogue and exploration. Subject positions can be regarded as ways of being that are influenced by the context within which we live. The approach described in this chapter draws upon psychodynamic theory, Freudian and Lacanian, and incorporates the approach to discourse described by Fairclough (1995), Gillett (1999) and Kaye (1999).

Discourses are ways of thinking, talking, acting and reacting within particular contexts that are accepted and understandable by others within the same culture. In other words, discourses allow what we say and do to be comprehensible to others. Within health and social care, these can include biomedical discourses, nursing discourses, caring discourses, psychological discourses, managerial discourses, lay discourses, disease discourses, and illness discourses. For example, biomedical discourses assume that illnesses are biologically rather than socially determined, that doctors have knowledge and authority, and that patients are relatively powerless. In contrast, illness discourses focus on patient experiences, including the meaning of illness, the complexity of living with illness, and the responses of the sick person's wider social network.

■ Theoretical background

Sigmund Freud (1915) developed the concept of the unconscious which is concerned with how intrapsychic conflict occurs between two drives — Eros (love) and Thanatos (death). The dynamic tension between these two drives and the anxiety produced by the individual's relationship with others lead to the development of ego defence mechanisms. These defence mechanisms provide temporary relief from anxiety-producing frustrations and become habitual. However, these anxiety-producing frustrations compound over time and persist in the unconscious. The unconscious, while not directly accessible to conscious processes, was considered by Freud to reveal itself in thoughts, dreams, behaviour, symptoms and relationships which are amenable to analysis and interpretation. The unconscious influences individuals' experiences of themselves and others and is established by the meanings attached to significant interactions and how new experiences are mediated. These meanings influence later behaviour and interactions without an individual being necessarily conscious of them. The unconscious plays itself out in the therapeutic alliance through transference and counter-transference processes.

This conceptualization of the unconscious was also explored by Lacan, who was particularly interested in the relationship of language and the unconscious. Lacan (1979) developed two important concepts to explain how the unconscious is formed: 'mirror image' and 'Name of the Father'. He utilizes the image of the mirror to explain how individuals learn to recognize themselves. This mirror image provides an illusion of something external to the subject that appears as both the subject and an illusion of the subject. This process moves the subject's interest outside himself or herself and provides a representation of the individual's separateness from others. Although still emotionally meshed with others, primarily the mother, the subject is given a visual representation of himself or herself as a distinct entity. This recognition of the image produces a transformation in the individual and alters the way in which they engage with others. The mirror image presents a sign of the self to the self, the significance of which is culturally determined. It provides a visual confirmation of the expectation that the self is distinct from others.

The second Lacanian concept that is useful in understanding the development of the unconscious is the 'Name of the Father' (Lacan, 1979). This represents the symbolic intrusion of their culture into the merged world of the mother and child. The 'Name of the Father' represents those cultural meanings that are permitted in a particular culture as determined by its language. Lacan employs the symbol of the phallus: 'I' as a symbol of the power of the 'Name of the Father'. It represents difference to the child in their separation from the mother and that identity is only achieved through loss and division. The 'Name of the Father' can be regarded as the voice of authority in relation to cultural norms.

In taking the 'Name of the Father' the child identifies particular attributes as the ideal. For the child to challenge this image of the ideal would be a cultural transgression. It is only possible to conceptualize a self as distinct from the culture in which it is situated because each self is constructed by its own unique experiences, yet also has experiences common to that culture. The individual is born into a culture that has already constituted potential culturally sanctioned subject positions (e.g. girl, boy, woman, man, mother, father). The performance of these subjects' positions is reinforced by others within the culture as 'normal'. This desire to be regarded as normal is reinforced by the unconscious desire to be recognised by others and to recognise others; to have relationships with others. It is the performance of this desire and the experience of its performance which provides both a point of difference and a point of connection between the self and the other. By understanding the ways in which language works we understand the processes of the psyche.

The role of cultural and social discourses is central to these Lacanian concepts and also to a discursive approach. Fairlcough (1995) describes language as a social and cultural process. Discourses have a constructive effect in shaping how we understand ourselves and others and how we act in relation to this. Of particular interest is the taken-for-granted and unquestioned ways that language is used to reproduce cultural and social norms. Gillett (1999) suggests that the history of each individual's exposure to different discourses is the history of their mind and personality due to the intimate relationship between brain function, biochemistry and sociocultural experiences. Throughout their lives individuals need to be able to participate in meaning-making and integrate conflicting meanings or discourses (Gillett, 1999). Relationships with others cue the individual to what is worth attending to; therefore words and their meanings have a formative effect on the contents of the mind and the connections that underpin psychic life. Meanings can shape or influence the microprocessing structure of the brain by setting up nodes or configurations of sensitivities to patterns of information and then forming connections between those functional nodes. Brain-processing is significantly shaped by words and their meanings as the neural networks register preferred excitation patterns associated with particular experiences.

Kaye (1999) suggests that a therapeutic alliance provides a context in which one connects with the experiential world of another and in which the other feels their world experience to be accepted and acknowledged as meaningful. He describes this as taking a 'receptive stance' that involves exploration of the person's perspective as well as prompting alternative constructions to emerge. He suggests that this is a generative and constructive process of meaning creation, which seeks to forge new understandings via the juxtaposition of multiple perspectives in conversational interchange – a process that involves the reinterpretation or resymbolisation of discourse (Kaye, 1999, p. 32). He proposes that a psychotherapeutic role involves reconceptualizing the individual's experience to facilitate the development of new meanings and possibilities. This involves responses that

- Bring the other to attend *to* rather than *from* their beliefs and presuppositions.
- Have the person explore their world from a new perspective.
- Prompt the emergence of new ways of construing experience and changed interpersonal attributes.
- Promote a questioning of the restraints imposed by beliefs that have been taken for granted as true.

The aim of this approach is to assist the person to establish some meaning around their mental distress and their experiences by exploring the discourses that have impacted on their current disabling understandings and finding alternative discourses that are more enabling. This involves helping the person to

1. Recognise the meaning of their current distress. This is the assessment phase of the psychotherapeutic process. The recognition of the nature of the person's distress can begin by seeking information about the person's feelings and relationships with others, particularly incidents in which their distress is triggered. This recognition is part of a psychotherapeutic process of recognising the person and accepting their narrative without taking on their frame of reference. From the information obtained during this process of engagement a clinical formulation can be developed that addresses the discursive, situational, psychodynamic and social processes influencing the person's health status and how these could be addressed. The formulation is therefore a way of understanding the person rather than attaching a label to their behaviour and feelings.

2. Make connections between the person's distress and the discourses that have impacted on this. This involves helping the person to put into words something that is often very painful and requires the development of a trusting alliance. This involves a trust in the health or social care worker's skills and their ability to contain strong outpourings of feelings. The establishment of connections also involves enabling the person to see how patterns from the past shape and give meaning to the present. Helping the person to establish connections involves helping the person to become aware of their communication style or how they respond in interaction with others. It also involves exploring the defensive responses that they may have utilized to hide or cope with their feelings. This awareness of communication patterns can assist the person to identify the ways of being (subject position) that they engage with in particular situations and evaluate the effectiveness of these.

3. Situate the person's experiences in a wider sociocultural context. The person can be assisted to explore their current experiences within the sociocultural context in which they have occurred. The sociocultural context values some subject positions more than others. Ways of being in the world that reflect the Western cultural norms of unitariness, rationality, productivity and moderation (Crowe, 2000) are those given more value in Western societies. Feelings of inadequacy, distress or helplessness may be reinforced when social problems are considered to be problems of faulty individual functioning. The person's sociocultural context determines how they can act and the options available to them. This phase involves raising questions about the values and beliefs that underpin the person's perspective of events to enable the person to begin their own questioning. This questioning can be used to explore how these culturally imposed values and beliefs may be contributing to or maintaining distressing feelings.

4. Promote an understanding of the potential for difference. This involves helping the person accept the potential for difference in the way they may experience or express themselves and how they could relate to others. In this phase of the alliance the person is encouraged to explore the expectations that they have of others and begin to hypothesise about what others may expect of them. The emphasis is on helping the person to develop the capacity to reflect on their own and others' behaviour and interactions.

5. Explore alternative subject positions (ways of being in the world) that are more satisfying and less problematic. This can provide the person with the opportunity to engage with different subject positions in their interactions with others. People have a range of subject positions from which they can respond to others. The performance of particular subject positions can be regarded as particular intersections of culture, gender,

class, and race. A sense of self is constituted by the repeated performance of particular subject positions and meaning is determined by
the subject positions to which people have access. The experimentation
with alternative subject positions within a supportive therapeutic alliance
allows for this creation of new meanings and understandings of the self
and alliances with others.

■ Example from practice

Below is a case scenario, divided into six sections and each followed by a
series of questions which will illustrate how this approach can be applied to
a person's situation:

Case study – Simon

Simon is a 28-year old male who is seeking treatment for depression for the first time. He describes becoming depressed about three
years ago following a back injury. At that time he was working in a
creative environment, had been married for one year, and had an
18-month-old son. Following his resignation from his job, he moved
cities and began working for his wife's family business doing clerical
work, which he found generally unsatisfying.

He is the oldest in a family with three siblings. When he was about
12 years old his mother left the family home because of domestic
violence, and he and his siblings were raised be their father, who
was physically abusive. Both parents had abused alcohol regularly
throughout Simon's childhood and when he was 17 years old Simon
attended treatment for his alcohol abuse.

Simon describes his mood as being low since moving cities but
lately it had been worsening with suicidal thoughts, poor sleep, inability to function competently in his job, and loss of motivation and
energy. His lower back continues to give him pain and he sees a physiotherapist regularly. He does not want to take medication but is eager
to receive therapy to address his problems.

☐ *Reflective exercise*

- What are the symptoms of depression and how can it occur?
- What might the relationship be between physical illness and depression?
- How does a person's social context influence how they feel about them?

- How does physical violence impact on children?
- How do social factors impact on a person's physical or mental health?

□ Recognising the distress

The initial process of engagement in establishing a therapeutic alliance involved taking a 'receptive stance' in order to connect with Simon's experiential world and acknowledge it as meaningful. This included instilling a sense of hope in the possibility of change while Simon was encouraged to talk about what he thought was the source of his distress. This process was not straightforward but involved Simon exploring a range of experiences he had found dissatisfying. Simon was encouraged to reflect on this and over the next few sessions he revealed that he thought he was 'not a proper man'. He was encouraged to explore in depth what he meant by 'proper man' and it emerged that this was associated with being a provider for his family, being able to protect his family, having a job that was valued, having his opinion valued, being a decision-maker, being respected and looked up to by others, having material possessions, and having interests similar to the other men in his wife's family. His inability to participate in many physical activities due to his lower back pain served to emphasise to him that he lacked the desirable attributes of masculinity.

When he was prompted to explore whether he was describing a particular man or an amalgamation of men he knew, Simon identified that he held his brother-in-law, his wife's sister's husband, to be the epitome of masculinity. This man was regarded by Simon as hard-working, had his own business, made lots of money, was respected by other family members, and was regarded as having considerable social prestige. It was pointed out to Simon that he might be idealising his brother-in-law and he was prompted to consider what he would gain or lose if he were to possess similar attributes. Initially Simon could only focus on how his life would improve if he were more like his brother-in-law but with consistent prompting he was able to identify that some of those attributes may not be personally satisfying. He realised that he would find his brother-in-law's occupation very unrewarding and it would diminish the time he had available to pursue his creative interests and his time with his family. Simon acknowledged that there were no material possessions that he could acquire from this occupation that he would find meaningful. However, this did not shift his perception of himself as not 'a proper man'.

□ *Reflective Exercise*

- Where do our understandings of masculinity and femininity come from?
- How do these understandings develop and become taken for granted?
- How do you see yourself as a woman or a man?

- How do you think you measure up to your culture's expectations for your gender?
- How do gendered norms impact on your choice of profession?

☐   Establishing connections

The establishment of connections involves enabling the person to see how patterns from the past shape and give meaning to the present. This involves exploring how apparently disconnected present-day experiences, behaviours, and feelings may be connected to past fears and anxieties. Chodorow (1999) suggests that this process enables what are initially experienced as discontinuities to come to be seen as continuous, with internal representations of the past and with each other. The exploration of relationship patterns helps the person to make connections between the feelings and the subject positions that they assume in their relation-ships with others. It involves making connections between how the person is currently feeling in relation to others and what has happened in past relationships. This may be done in the psychotherapeutic relationship by identifying patterns as they are described and questioning the repetition of these. It was noted that whenever Simon made a statement regarding his lack of self-worth and low mood he had linked this to how he was evaluating his worth against a particular construction of masculinity.

Kaye (1999) suggests that the discursive approach avoids taking on the person's frame of reference as the sole explanation of experiences but takes a position that he describes as a 'superordinate framework'. This involves responding to the person's narrative and recontextualising it to help facili-tate new meanings and new possibilities. The recontextualisation provides the opportunity for making new connections between how the person is feeling and their experiences and beliefs:

> The shift in perspective serves to highlight previously unnoticed connec-tions between behaviour events, beliefs and feelings as well as to disrupt previously automatic behaviour sequences.
>
> (Kaye, 1999, p. 23)

With Simon this involved not buying into the meanings he associated with his lifestyle, the options available to him, or his perceptions of himself or others. Simon was helped to make some new connections by becoming aware of his communication style with others in which he often withdrew or conceded to others despite having beliefs to the contrary. The identification of these patterns of communication helped Simon to make connections between what he did and how he felt. This awareness of communication pat-terns assisted Simon to identify the subject positions with which he engaged in particular situations and to evaluate the effectiveness and satisfaction associated with them.

> Simon identified that he had never really thought about his sense of who he was as a man until the birth of his son. This birth had a strong impact on how he viewed himself and the permanence of the relationships between him, his wife, and his child. He had had a sense that he really had 'to get it right' – be the best father, be the best husband. It emerged that the work pressures at his previous job were related to trying to balance a family life with a work life that had long hours and a large social component. He felt he had to make a decision to get out of his job in order to participate in his family in the way that he thought was the right way. The result of this was dissatisfaction with himself and with his inability to perform his role in the family and his new job that was more amenable to family life.
>
> Simon was encouraged to explore the history of his perception of 'being a proper man'. He eventually revealed that all his ideals were based on not being like his father. Thus his father acted as a reference point for all that Simon did not want to be and he had constructed a sense of self that could not tolerate any similarities with his father. Simon had never made this connection before and was quite shocked when he articulated it as he thought he had disconnected his feelings from his father and had taken a pitying stance towards him when he talked about him.
>
> He did not feel anger towards his father but rather a sense of repulsion and a fear that he may become like him. Simon's anger was directed mostly towards his mother for abandoning him and his siblings. He was surprised that he still felt anger towards her because he thought that he had dealt with this in his alcohol treatment and that he had moved on to forgiveness. Mostly, however, Simon felt angry with himself for not meeting his own expectations of masculinity. Simon's sense of self reflected the Lacanian contention that individuals project their experiences on an image of the self which is regarded as fixed. This image was referenced to others and reflected how he perceived he was identified by others.

☐   *Reflective Exercise*

- When you imagine yourself what image is produced?
- How does this image of yourself impact on your relationships with others?
- What defence mechanism are you prone to utilise when this image of yourself is threatened?
- What defence mechanisms do you employ when confronted with unfamiliar situations?

☐   Situating the distress in its sociocultural context

Simon was prompted to consider the social and cultural factors that influenced his construction of manhood. He was able to recognise that the image of a man that he was upholding was part of the dominant discourse on masculinity. What Simon was exploring was the Lacanian claim that when the individual takes up a position as 'I' this represents a cultural intrusion into what had been a merged experience with his mother. The phallus represented the meanings for masculinity that were permitted in language. Simon had taken up two different cultural representations of masculinity and was upholding one as the ideal and the other as its opposite. After exploring what this meant for him and for other men, Simon was encouraged to identify other possible performances of masculinity.

Kaye (1999, p. 34) suggested that a discursive approach involves working towards exploring the dominant sociocultural discursive formations and associated practices by which a person is positioned. Within the psychotherapeutic alliance questions can be raised about the values and beliefs that underpin the person's self-image to enable the person to begin their own questioning. This questioning can be used to explore how these culturally imposed values and beliefs may be contributing to or maintaining the depression.

The psychotherapeutic alliance helped Simon to contextualise his feelings and responses by helping him to retell his experiences in a way that reconstructed the experience as socially and culturally situated. The factors which were beyond his control were identified and he was able to identify possibilities for change.

☐   *Reflective Exercise*

• Which cultural norms have the biggest impact on how you perceive yourself?
• How does your culture impact on your experience of being a student?
• How does your culture define the attributes of normality?
• How does your culture define the attributes of abnormality?
• What behaviours do you consider unacceptable from a cultural perspective?
• What discourses influence your understandings of health and social work?

☐   Promoting the acceptance of difference

Simon was encouraged to explore other possibilities for masculine subject positions. This was done by encouraging him to note representations of masculinity both in the media and in his interactions with other men. Role-play was used to assist Simon in finding more satisfying responses to others that did not confine him to the idealised representation of masculinity that was associated with his brother-in-law and the spurned representation associated with his father.

In this process Simon was also able to identify positive aspects in his father and how he believed that his father probably also experienced tensions related to what he felt he was expected to do as a man and the need to bring up three children. While Simon regarded his father as unsuccessful in this role he was able to acknowledge his father's positive attributes and the lack of preparation his father probably had for childcare, which he generally regarded as women's work:

> Simon hypothesised that his father probably felt ashamed and out of his depth in bringing up children and that he was probably dealing with his own issues. Simon was able to begin to identify that he had developed a polarised view of the subject positions associated with masculinity. For Simon this impasse was tied up with how he thought of himself as a man and how he perceived others thought about him. He felt trapped and could conceive of no way to resolve this because he considered his depression to be another sign of his inadequacy as a man.

The effect of this on Simon was that he was able to position his father as a not totally negative role model while also acknowledging the distressing experiences that Simon had been through. Effectively Simon was able to tolerate an ambivalent attitude towards both his father and his brother-in-law. He could identify a representation of both men that acknowledged strengths and weaknesses in their performances of masculine subject positions. He acknowledged that there were multiple ways that he could 'be a proper man' and that there were alternative subject positions that he could explore. An important aspect of this process involved helping Simon to manage ambiguity and the contradictions associated with masculinity in our society.

☐   Exploring alternative subject positions

Because Simon could articulate a tolerance for difference, he began putting some of these ideas into practice. Simon was provided with the opportunity within the psychotherapeutic alliance to engage with different subject positions in his interactions with others. These subject positions can be regarded as those modes of being that constitute a sense of self. People have a range of subject positions from which they can respond to others. The performance of particular subject positions can be regarded as particular intersections of culture, gender, class, and race. A sense of self is constituted by the repeated performance of particular subject positions and meaning is determined by the subject positions to which people have access. The meanings that can be attributed to subject positions are developed through relations with others and the experiences of acceptance or rejection. The subject positions when depressed may reinforce the symptoms:

> Simon was encouraged to try alternative subject positions that challenged old assumptions about himself in relation to others. He was encouraged to engage in these subject positions outside the psychotherapeutic relation in his everyday life. With practice and support Simon gradually reconstructed an image of himself that was less disabling and more emotionally fulfilling. He started to commence some creative projects at home and gradually developed more confidence in himself until he decided to resign from his boring job and seek more creative opportunities. The work he produced was highly regarded by future employers and after six months he entered part-time employment and occupied the rest of his time by becoming the main childcare provider and developing new projects.

The experimentation with alternative subject positions within the support of the psychotherapeutic alliance allowed for the creation of alternative meanings of masculinity for Simon. It allowed for challenging, in a supportive manner, the beliefs that underpinned his actions in relation to others and encouraging the practice of new strategies. It provided Simon with a consistent source of affirmation and facilitated the development of an image of himself as a competent, creative person capable of meaningful and rewarding relations with others.

Reflective Exercise
- Are your personal and professional values congruent?
- How do you manage situations when a professional obligation may not be congruent with your personal values?
- What aspects of yourself in relation to practising within your profession would you like to develop further?
- What discourses could you draw on to implement these developments?

■ Conclusion

From a discursive approach the therapeutic alliance can focus on new significance in the individual's experience in a way that provides them with a sense of meaning and agency in their life. This involves being aware of how discourses impact on how we construct ourselves and our relationships with others. In the therapeutic alliance it involves actively assisting the individual to recognise the symbolic meaning embedded in their language and behaviour and the role that language plays in constructing their experiences; helping the individual to recognise the taken-for-granted meanings in their cultural context; promoting difference and multiplicity in the individual's response to their social world; and facilitating the development of alternative subject positions that are more meaningful and satisfying. In order to be able to do this in a genuine and respectful manner we first need to be aware of how we can implement these strategies in our own lives.

References

Chodorow, N. (1999). *The Power of Feelings*. New Haven, CT: Yale University Press.

Crowe, M. (2000). Constructing normality: A discourse analysis of the Gillett, G. (1999). *The Mind and its Discontents*. Oxford: Oxford University Press.

Fairclough, N. (1995). *Critical Discourse Analysis*. London: Longman.

Kaye, J. (1999). Towards a non-regulative practice. In I. Parker (ed.), *Deconstructing Psychotherapy* (pp. 19–38). London: Sage.

Lacan, J. (1979). *The Four Fundamental Concepts of Psycho-Analysis (Trans by Alan Sheridan)*. Harmondsworth: Penguin.

Chapter 7

The voice of experience: Consumer perspective in the classroom

Brenda Happell and Cath Roper

■ Introduction

This chapter presents the case for consumer participation in the education of health care professionals and how the attitudes of professionals can be influenced by the active inclusion of consumers of health services in the education process. This chapter takes a very practical approach, describing an innovative and effective approach to capturing 'the voice of experience' as an integral part of the educational experience for mental health nurses with the powerful and valuable resource of a consumer academic.

■ Consumer perspective in the education of health care professionals

The provision of quality health care depends on professional practice with the specific aim of meeting the needs of those people who use those services. These people are generally known as patients, clients, consumers or users. For the purposes of this chapter we have used 'consumer' as it is the term most commonly used in mental health services in Australia. The contents of this chapter are not limited to consumers of mental health services and are likely to have a much broader relevance. However, the consumer movement has been led from the mental health field, and the discrimination and disempowerment of consumers is felt most markedly in this arena (Middleton, Stanton and Renouf, 2004).

To many readers it may appear perfectly logical that as health care is about those who consume services, the views and experiences of consumers should be central to the education of health professionals. It is likely that few would disagree, but it is the way in which we ensure that professional education reflects consumer needs and wishes that may be an issue of dispute (Happell, 2007). Those responsible for the education of health and social care professionals may believe the programmes they teach do indeed reflect consumer experience because of the substantial clinical experience of the academic staff. They may well believe that the lessons learned and expertise gained brings 'the voice of experience' into the classroom.

We do not dispute the value of this approach but argue that on its own it is insufficient. Developing health professionals with the skills, attitudes and sensitivities required to provide high quality and individually based care and treatment requires 'consumer perspective in the classroom'. However, 'in the classroom' must be interpreted in its broader sense. In order that consumer perspective is truly reflected in what is taught, the voice of consumers must not be limited to the classroom. Rather consumers should contribute to shaping professional education at all levels through active involvement in all stages including curriculum design, teaching, assessment and evaluation (Warne and McAndrew, 2004). 'The voice of experience' must be genuine and not reflect the tokenistic principles that threaten to dilute the emancipatory potential of consumer participation in professional education.

■ The context for the consumer academic role

During the year 2000, an academic position for a consumer of mental health services was developed and implemented in a psychiatric nursing centre in Melbourne, Australia. This position was the first known of its kind in the world in any discipline or any health care setting.

In mental health, the inclusion of consumer perspective in the education and preparation of mental health practitioners is recognised through policy directives. (Commonwealth Department of Health, 2003; Commonwealth Department of Health and Ageing, 2003; Deakin Human Services, 1999; Department of Health, 2005; Department of Human Services, Victoria, 2002). From an international perspective, a policy goal of the National Health Service in the United Kingdom is to develop mental health services that reflect the individual needs of consumers. An increased ability to participate in all aspects of mental health services is considered the key to ensuring its success (Department of Health, 2005). In the United States consumer and carer participation is not so clearly embedded in written policy. The Department of Health and Human Services and Centre for Mental Health established the Consumer Affairs Program, developed to enhance and support meaningful participation in mental health services (Substance Abuse and Mental Health Services Administration, n.d.).

In Australia, most disciplines preparing students for working in health and social care in undergraduate and postgraduate courses would include at least a session delivered by consumers and carers. Epstein and Shaw (1997) delineate three types of education effort: leaf work, branch work and root work.

Leaf sessions are one-off. For example, a consumer might come into a class and talk about his or her experience of madness, or of using cancer care services, or being unable to access respite services. Students often find these to be significant, memorable and powerful sessions. But the question remains: how do such sessions influence attitudes, practice and service delivery?

Root work is systemic. It is long-term and developmental. It requires the building of relationships and formal/informal structures that will sustain consumer perspective. Branch work would describe activities occurring as a result of the relationships that form the 'root system', such as auditing existing curricula, involvement in teaching, staff selection, developing assessment tasks, marking student work, sustained and progressive delivery of content, team teaching throughout a subject, and training health and social care practitioners in interview skills.

The implementation of the consumer academic position reflected acknowledgement that leaf work is not likely to make a profound and long-term impact on the attitudes of health professionals, and that indeed it ran the risk of being tokenistic and exploitative of consumer experience and knowledge. In the example above, it is not uncommon once the consumer has left the classroom after relaying a personal account that the students are asked to identify symptoms or consider a likely diagnosis, thus undermining and devaluing the human experience into what we might refer to as scientific knowledge (Warne and McAndrew, 2007). The aim of the consumer academic position was to move beyond the leaves to develop the roots, and ultimately allow branches to grow and flourish.

■ Why the title 'consumer academic'?

The use of this title has been unexpectedly controversial (Happell, Pinikahana and Roper, 2002). People have often asked us why we include consumer in the title, suggesting that this amounts to labelling and is therefore potentially discriminatory (Happell, Pinikahana and Roper, 2002). Indeed it was suggested by the reviewer of a journal article we wrote that 'consumer' should be removed from the title to avoid this discrimination.

Given that the aim of the position was to facilitate consumer perspective within psychiatric nursing academia, it was considered essential to promote the fact that a consumer held this position. The first essential recruitment criteria were being a consumer of mental health services and having an active involvement in the consumer movement. That is, she was specifically employed for her consumer background. It is difficult to understand how this innovative approach could be actively promoted and at the same time avoiding public acknowledgement of consumer status.

In response to the reviewer's comment the consumer academic wrote a preface to the article (Happell, Pinikahana and Roper, 2002) to explain the origins of the term and the reasons why she chose this title to describe her position:

> It has been a matter of pride that the title also explicitly states it is a 'consumer' role – reflecting a distinctive consumer perspective. It is this all too infrequently heard perspective that makes the role unique (p. 240).

■ A unique role and a unique subject

Since the inception of this position, the consumer academic has delivered consumer perspective content into the postgraduate education for nurses choosing to specialise in the mental health field. In the initial stages, this consisted of 16 hours of face-to-face teaching spread across two existing subjects. Evaluations of this initiative showed that consumer perspective in the classroom was both valued by students and found to positively influence their attitudes towards consumer participation in mental health care (Happell and Roper, 2003).

At the beginning of 2007, some six years after the introduction of the consumer academic position, the roots had strengthened and enhanced the growth of many new branches. One of these was the introduction of a core subject entitled 'Consumer Perspective and Participation'. This is a full subject consisting of 36 hours of face-to-face teaching. The curricula has been developed and delivered with the involvement of a range of consumers, with the consumer academic as the subject co-ordinator.

The consumer academic has herself experienced involuntary detention and treatment annually over a 13-year period. She identifies as using a survivor perspective and this is made transparent to students from the first session which introduces the consumer movement, its history and concerns. Survivor perspective refers to having survived the mental health service system, rather than the specific mental illness:

> A survivor perspective engages a critical eye to service use as directly experienced. Like related human rights movements, survivor perspective is typically concerned with citizenship, equality, self-determination, social justice and pride in being who we are.
>
> (Happell et al., 2008)

■ Education purpose

The subject is based on a 'critical consumer perspective' approach. Among the assumptions informing this approach are the following:

- Consumer perspective authenticates the 'lay' knowledge we all have about the well-being of ourselves and our communities.
- Hearing directly from consumers is 'first-person' knowledge, which can be gained in no other way.
- Social and cultural factors are important to understand for their causal and consequential role in people's well-being.
- Bio-psychiatric approaches to care should be critiqued and understood as only one body of knowledge.
- Health and social care practitioners should understand the impact of legislation on consumers and on their relationships with consumers.
- A key skill for all health professionals is the ability to critically reflect on one's role, workplace, the health and social care system, and wider social culture.

■ Delivery

The consumer perspective subject is composed of four modules: critical perspectives; models of care; consumer involvement in treatment; and consumer involvement in service reform. Each module is composed of three sessions of three hours' duration. Discussion, brainstorming and small group activities are the main learning methods used.

Student debates are used to stimulate discussion and allow students to experience 'occupying the teaching space'. This means they are able to nominate content that is of interest to them, such as 'the mental health act should be abolished' or 'de-institutionalisation has failed'.

Guest consumer tutors with expertise in particular areas such as consumer consultancy, poetry, art and activism are invited into the class. Consumers are also welcome to sit in on the classes in an observer capacity. This structure has been chosen because student feedback suggests the approach to be both useful and enjoyable.

■ Assessment tasks

Assessment tasks were developed with the assistance of three additional consumer educators who were also involved in curricula planning. For the first assessment, students are asked to articulate what they give value to by investigating an approach to care that reflects these principles, using both a consumer and a non-consumer reference. Students are then asked to critically reflect on what supports or impedes this approach to care. The feedback collected to date suggests that many students welcomed the opportunity to think about what personal principles govern their practice and indicated that they had not had the opportunity to do so elsewhere. For others, it highlighted the conflict between how they would ideally like to practice and the working environment, which sometimes prevents the ideal from becoming a reality.

The second assessment explores the difference between substitute and supported decision-making. Substitute refers to those decisions made on behalf of the consumer and believed to be in his or her best interest whether or not he or she would agree. Supported decision-making involves understanding individual wishes and preferences and assisting consumers to make their own health care decisions.

Students are asked to describe an example from their clinical practice where a consumer was subject to substitute decision-making. Students are then asked to consider how a supported decision-making model could have been applied, and what different outcomes there might have been for all involved. The assignment asks students to reflect on the impact of substitute decision-making on the consumer and thus on their clinical practice, and then allows students to explore other models which are centred on maximising the self-determination of the consumer and which require different clinical skills.

■ The proof of the pudding is in the eating: Examples from practice

The best way to picture how consumer experience and perspective can be brought into the classroom would be to be there. Since this is not possible for most readers, the next best thing is to read about and reflect on a written description. The following provides an example of the content, process and activities associated with a selected part of the curriculum.

☐ The culture of psychiatry

☐ *Description of the session*

This is the last session in the first module called 'Critical Perspectives'. The session begins with students reporting back on homework. In the previous session they were asked to observe how staff they work with handle their interactions with consumers and the impact that modelling good or bad practice might have. The session introduces the idea that social or cultural realities are an observable phenomenon that can be described, that have an impact on us, and that we in turn impact upon (Ivbijaro, Kolkiewicz and Palazidou, 2005). The session has three parts.

Part one
Learning objectives

- To develop an awareness of culture as a phenomenon.
- To understand and consider the impact of discrimination, prejudice and labelling.

1. Examining elements of culture

The underlying theme in this session is the power of social phenomena. Three controversial figures, namely Solomon Asch (n.d.), Stanley Milgram (1997) and Jane Elliot (n.d.), and their work in the areas of conformity, obedience and discrimination, respectively, are introduced. There are usually a couple of students who will have encountered these figures before, so the session begins with students offering what they already know.

The basic outlines of the research of Asch (n.d.) and Milgram (1997) and the workshops of Elliot (n.d.) are then presented. In the 1950s Asch, a pioneering social psychologist, designed an experiment in which test subjects were asked to perform a simple exercise. 'Actors' and a test subject were each asked to determine which of three lines on a diagram was the longest. The test subject gave their answer after the 'actors'. There was no ambiguity about what the 'correct' answer was, and the actors were instructed to give 'incorrect' answers. Only 29 percent of the test subjects were prepared to go against the majority, even though they were upset by the difference between what they saw as the 'right' answer and the answers given first by the others in the room.

Milgram (1997) conducted experiments in which an 'actor' was involved in a simple word game while the 'test' subject was instructed to deliver electric shocks if the person took too long to answer, or was incorrect. The researcher told the subject to administer a shock, starting at low voltage and rising to 450 volts.

Milgram (1997) found that 65 percent of his subjects were prepared to deliver shocks of up to 450 volts, even where there was great protest from the 'actor', because a scientific authority told them they were required to. These controversial experiments showed a human propensity to conform to a perceived authority figure, even when it involved doing something 'inhumane' to another person.

The 'blue eyes/brown eyes' workshops of Elliot (n.d.) offer participants the opportunity to understand how culture is experienced differently by those who are privileged and those who are discriminated against. Elliot's essential point is that those who belong to the powerful group (white) benefit, even if indirectly, from that power. In this context, only the powerful could argue that discrimination does not exist, and only those not directly affected by discrimination can remain blind to its effects.

Students are shocked about both the design and the findings of Asch's and Milgram's research experiments, leading to discussion about research ethics and whether or not this kind of research could take place today. 'Peer pressure', obedience to authority and examining discrimination are backdrops to moving more closely towards an examination of psychiatry itself as a phenomenon.

2. Brainstorm: How would you describe the culture of psychiatry?

This activity invites students to call out descriptions, which are noted on the whiteboard. Words like 'paternalistic', 'diagnoses', 'disease-based', 'black humour', 'hierarchical', 'medical', 'containment', 'coercion' cover the whiteboard. Usually it takes about ten minutes before some students realise there are very few, if any, positive words. That usually leads to a reinvigoration of new words like 'care', 'listening', 'respect', 'recovery'. In past years this activity has been cathartic in that students can externalise all the features they identify as 'getting on the road' of how they want to practise. When they see a collective description, covering a whiteboard, they are able to see that there are some things they have no control over and others they do. They also see that they have built a characterisation of a phenomenon that is separate from the self. There needs to be a break before proceeding to the next activity so that it appears to be unconnected.

Part two
1. **Discussion: My adolescence**

The discussion turns to the following questions:

- **How does our culture present adolescence** (e.g. on TV programmes, in the news, by previous generations, as consumers of goods targeted by advertising)? Is puberty occurring earlier these days? Are kids becoming adolescents at younger age?
- **What are our different cultural beliefs about adolescence** (e.g. the status of turning 21, turning 13, cross-cultural beliefs about adolescence)?

2. Activity: What were you like as an adolescent?

For this activity, students are divided into pairs. They tell stories to each other about what they were like as an adolescent. Where students are engaged in pair work they know that in feeding back they will provide their partner's response, not their own. This models careful listening in class work and also builds the intimacy of the group.

During the feedback session the students provide a couple of words or phrases about their partners. These are written on the whiteboard in a column with a blank column next to it. Students find this fun because they get to know the person next to them in a way they haven't previously. There is laughing and joking as people reveal that they were a 'wild child' or a 'party animal' or a 'goody goody'.

After all students have reported back, two volunteers are asked to come to the whiteboard with a marker. The teacher asks the rest of the group to provide the medical or pathological equivalent of these words and phrases. These are recorded in the blank column next to the descriptor. This part of the session is quick and energetic, and again, students are laughing, some laughing and cringing at the same time. Pretty soon, the second column is filled with words like 'isolating', 'manic', 'elevated', 'dual diagnosis'.

As the activity finishes, the teaching objective is very clear, without need for any explanation. We contemplate the lists and intuitively understand several things: that labels are reductive, they take away the story of the person, they carry with them all kinds of other meanings, they do not reveal what we are like as people. We discuss feelings associated with this activity and move on to looking at the implications for practice and the question 'Does it make any difference to how you view someone once you know their "label"?'

3. Reading in class

A volunteer reads the poem 'You and Me' by Debbie Sesula (www.power2u.org). The reading is followed by an invitation to respond openly to the content in any way students wish.

You and Me
If you're overly excited
You're happy
If I'm overly excited
I'm manic.
If you imagine the phone ringing
You're stressed out
If I imagine the phone ringing
I'm psychotic.
If you're crying and sleeping all day
You're sad and need time out
If I'm crying and sleeping all day
I'm depressed and need to get up.
If you're afraid to leave your house at night
You're cautious

If I'm afraid to leave my house at night
I'm paranoid.
If you speak your mind and express your opinions
You're assertive
If I speak my mind and express my opinions
I'm aggressive.
If you don't like something and mention it
You're being honest
If I don't like something and mention it
I'm being difficult.
If you get angry
You're considered upset
If I get angry
I'm considered dangerous.
If you over-react to something
You're sensitive
If I over-react to something
I'm out of control.
If you don't want to be around others
You're taking care of yourself and relaxing
If I don't want to be around others
I'm isolating myself and avoiding.
If you talk to strangers
You're being friendly
If I talk to strangers
I'm being inappropriate.
For all of the above you're not told to take a pill or are hospitalized, *but I am!*

4. Reflective questions

- How might conformity, obedience and discrimination be useful in understanding the culture of psychiatry?
- How does the culture of the workplace impact on practitioners and the people they care for?
- How can you have an impact on your work culture?
- Can you know a culture if you are inside it?

☐ *Part three – The social model of disability*

After a break the session continues with the following objectives, encouraging students to

- Appreciate the difference between medical and social models of disability.
- Apply understandings of facilitative/obstructive factors in environment.

Table 7.1 The social model of disability framework from the consumer viewpoint

Experienced factors		Enabling	Disabling
Physical	Effects of medications.	Can contribute to stability.	Can have serious physical health implications.
Social	Separate services for people diagnosed with psychiatric illness.	Can give a sense of belonging and safety.	Maintains separation and might contribute to feeling 'lesser'.
Attitudinal	Media.	Can be used to lobby for the concerns consumers have.	Can focus on the dangerousness of consumers and contribute to community fears.

Students are introduced to the medical and social models of disability. The social model describes disability as an experienced phenomenon (Birmingham Government, 2007; Happell, 2007). The 'disability' describes the relationship of the person to external environmental factors (Birmingham Government, 2007; Happell, 2007). This is very different from the conception of a psychiatric disability being a 'problem' that a person has, stemming from an 'illness' that prevents them from being 'normal'. A social model of disability encourages exploration of the impact of environmental factors like poverty, discrimination, access to resources, equity on people's well-being. In this model, environmental factors are divided into three categories: physical, social and attitudinal (Table 7.1). These factors are experienced as either facilitative or obstructive by an individual or group.

The final part of the session is designed to adapt the framework to give students a way to analyse workplace culture and broader culture.

We go back to the whiteboard with the collective student descriptions of psychiatry as a culture. Firstly, students decide whether the environmental features identified are physical, social or attitudinal. Then they assess whether each feature is enabling or disabling of the way they want to practice.

This is done as a whole group exercise on the whiteboard in a grid like the one shown in Table 7.2. Through this activity students are further able to externalise and describe what they are experiencing in their work.

By describing, acknowledging and externalising some of the features of psychiatric culture, students can identify many obstacles they cannot change. However, they can also see potential enablers. Education, seeking good role models, accessing supervision, being grounded in one's own principles, finding 'kindred' peers, advocating when needed are all things

Table 7.2 The framework applied to the culture of psychiatry from student viewpoint

Experienced factors		Enabling	Disabling
Physical	Use of seclusion and restraint.	Can contribute to stabilising ward.	Can have serious traumatic impact.
Social	Not 'breaking ranks' with your peers.	Can give you a sense of belonging/ security.	Can mean that bad practice goes unchecked.
Attitudinal	Black humour.	Helps you cope.	Could lead to cynicism and interfere with sense of compassion.

that students raise as empowering. This is an important place to leave the session by encouraging a realistic sense of how they might achieve change and in which areas, as well as how they might best take care of their own well-being.

■ Ingredients for a successful consumer academic position

Being the first of a kind offers the opportunity for innovation and creativity but limits the capacity to learn from the experience of others. Reflecting on the success of the consumer academic position led to the identification of four factors as crucial for the successful implementation of consumer perspective in the education of health and social care professionals:

- Partnership and commitment.
- Support.
- Scope.
- Autonomy.

☐ Partnership and commitment

If consumer perspective is to be genuine and effective, active involvement in the education process is a necessity. The professional members of the team must commit to working with consumers as partners. Involvement must begin with inception of the idea, to enable consumers to work on equal footing towards a shared vision.

The consumer academic position described in this chapter developed from a partnership between an academic centre and a consumer organisation. The partnership was formed at the beginning of the process and remained throughout. Importantly, equal numbers of consumers and health professionals were included in the project team. The partnership took collective responsibility for all stages of the recruitment process. The consumer academic joined the team following her appointment, meaning that consumers now outnumbered the health professionals. Without demonstrating this level of commitment, the initiative runs the risk of being tokenistic and therefore ineffective.

☐ Support

The academics reading this chapter may well remember the adjustments they needed to make when entering the realm of the higher education system. It is also likely that they will remember the benefits of peer support and mentorship. Academic and educational roles for consumers are still very much in their infancy, which limits the extent to which they may benefit from collegiality and professional identity (Happell and Roper, 2006).

Consumers need the opportunity to interact with and be supported by a broader group of consumers. This may be achieved through, for example, a project or advisory team with strong consumer membership where the consumer academic can brainstorm ideas and receive feedback or listen to the suggestions of other members. Formal supervision with a consumer, preferably with experience as an academic or educator, should also be provided on a regular basis.

☐ Scope

If the aim of the position is to positively influence the attitudes of health and social care professionals, the consumer academic must be granted the scope to do so and it is important that the role is not restricted to teaching alone. An active role in curriculum development, student assessment and evaluative strategies (as described earlier in this chapter) is crucial to avoiding tokenism and ensuring that consumer perspective can move beyond leaf work to root and branch work.

Research and consultancy also provide important opportunities for consumer academics to contribute to the development and dissemination of knowledge, and to ensure that the consumer voice permeates the discourse of health and social care professionals at a number of levels.

Providing scope, while essential, presents its own challenges. Until consumer academics are present in large numbers, the breadth of the role will be limited, not by imagination but by reality. The implementation of a sole position cannot avoid the frustration of wanting the consumer to be involved in a multitude of projects, be a member of key committees, sit on interview panels, be an active researcher and teacher, and provide consultancy to services about enhancing consumer participation; in other words, wanting one person to fill the shoes of many. The consumer academic can run the risk of being 'burnt out' by unreasonable demands.

☐ Autonomy

Autonomy is the key to avoiding tokenism. The aim of the position is to provide voice to consumer perspective; then this voice must be respected. If the consumer academic needs to seek approval from his or her line manager before expressing an opinion, accepting an invitation to speak or to sit on a key committee, then autonomy is lost and the position runs the risk of being a superficial attempt at political correctness. Easier said than done. It is one thing to support the importance of autonomy but another to be prepared to defend it. Unfortunately, paternalistic attitudes prevail and many health and social care professionals are likely to feel challenged, even offended by the words or activities of a consumer academic (Roper and Happell, 2007). We experienced this professional defensiveness on a number of occasions. For example, the consumer academic was to produce a book of transcribed conversations between service receivers regarding their experiences of psychiatric nursing and the mental health service system (Roper, 2003). While by no means a universal response, some readers felt that nursing was attacked in the book and that there was a strong bias towards negative experiences with nurses.

Interestingly, though, the criticism on this and other occasions was not directed to the consumer academic herself but rather to her line manager, a nurse academic, with the suggestion that the final document should have been approved and to some degree censured. However, to do so would effectively make a mockery of this position. If consumer perspective is sought then consumer perspective must be accepted, warts and all, and not only when it produces what the health and social care professionals want to hear. Consumer academics and educators need to be able to work with the knowledge and confidence that their work will be valued, supported and, where necessary, defended.

☐ Reflective exercise

For those of you interested in implementing a consumer academic position please consider the following:

- The aims and potential benefits you would hope to see from this position.
- The extent to which your organisation is able to meet the essential criteria for success.

- Partnership and commitment.
- Support.
- Scope.
- Autonomy.
- The modifications that may need to be made to ensure the above factors are realised and sustainable.
- The strategies within your organisation and professional group that are likely to facilitate the implementation of a consumer academic position.
- The barriers within your organisation and professional group that are likely to impede the implementation of a consumer academic position.
- The ways in which you might strengthen the strategies and minimise the barriers.
- The potential funding sources for the consumer academic position.

■ Conclusion

If we start from the premise that consumer participation is an essential part of quality education for health professionals, the issue moves beyond why and becomes about how to implement such a role. This chapter has provided an overview of the introduction and development of the consumer academic role and a snapshot of the innovative educational approach and techniques she uses to familiarise students with the consumer perspective. As the result of our experience with this role, we developed some principles to guide the implementation of this position and these have been briefly described.

As a final word, we are extremely proud of this position and the achievements it has made. Our main regret is that similar positions are not commonplace within professional education. We hope this chapter provides some motivation to others to follow the path.

References

Asch, S. (n.d.). Solomon Asch experiment (1958) A Study of Conformity. Retrieved August 2007 from: http://www.age-of-the-sage.org/psychology/social/asch_conformity.html

Birmingham Government (2007). http://www.birmingham.gov.uk/GenerateContent?CONTENT_ITEM_ID=1196&CONTENT_ITEM_TYPE=0&MENU_ID=1815

Commonwealth Department of Health (2003). *National Practice Standards for Mental Health Practitioners.* Canberra: Commonwealth of Australia.

Commonwealth Department of Health and Ageing (2003). *Second National Mental Health Plan.* Canberra: Commonwealth of Australia.

Department of Human Services, Victoria (2002). *New Directions for Victoria's Mental Health Services.* Melbourne: Department of Human Services.

Deakin Human Services (1999). *Learning Together: Education and Training Partnerships in Mental Health Services.* Commonwealth Department of Health and Aged Care, Australian Government.

Department of Health (2005). *Creating a Patient-Led NHS: Delivering The NHS Improvement Plan.* London: Department of Health.

Elliot, J. (n.d.). Jane Elliot's Blue Eyes Brown Eyes Experiment. Retrieved August 2007 from: http://www.janeelliott.com/

Epstein, M. and Shaw, J. (1997). *Developing Effective Consumer Participation in Mental Health Services.* Melbourne: VMIAC.

Happell, B. (2007). 'We are all consumers of mental health services.' The hidden danger of promoting 'sameness'. *International Journal of Mental Health Nursing,* 16(3), 145–146.

Happell, B., Cowin, L., Roper, C., Foster, K. and McMaster, R. (2008). *Introducing Mental Health Nursing: A Consumer Oriented Approach.* Sydney: Allen and Unwin.

Happell, B., Pinikahana, J. and Roper, C. (2002). Attitudes of postgraduate nursing students towards consumer participation in mental health services and the role of the consumer academic. *International Journal of Mental Health Nursing,* 11(4), 240–250.

Happell, B. and Roper, C. (2006). The myth of representation: The case for consumer leadership. *The Australian e-Journal for the Advancement of Mental Health,* 5(3), Retrieved January 2007 from http://www.auseinet.com/journal/vol5iss3/happell.pdf

Happell, B. and Roper, C. (2003). The role of a mental health consumer in the education of postgraduate psychiatric nursing students: The students' evaluation. *Journal of Psychiatric & Mental Health Nursing,* 10(3), 343–350.

Ivbijaro, G.O., Kolkiewicz, L.A. and Palazidou, E. (2005). Mental health in primary care: Ways of working – the impact of culture. *Primary Care Mental Health,* 3(1), 47–53.

Middleton, P., Stanton, P. and Renouf, N. (2004). Consumer consultants in mental health services: Addressing the challenges. *Journal of Mental Health,* 13(5), 507–518.

Milgram, S. (1997). *Obedience to Authority: An Experimental View.* London: Pinter & Martin.

Roper, C. (ed.) (2003). *Sight Unseen – Conversations between Service Receivers On Mental Health Nursing and the Psychiatric Service System,* Carlton: CPNRP, University of Melbourne.

Roper, C. and Happell, B. (2007). Reflection without shame, reflection without blame: Towards a more collaborative understanding between mental health consumers and nurses. *Journal of Psychiatric and Mental Health Nursing,* 14(1), 85–91.

Warne, T. and McAndrew, S. (2007). Passive patient or engaged expert? using a ptolemaic approach to enhance mental health nurse education and practice. *International Journal of Mental Health Nursing,* 16(4), 224–229.

Warne, T. and McAndrew, S. (eds) (2004). *Using Patient Experience in Nurse Education.* Palgrave: London.

Chapter 8

The potential of literature and poetry

Ann Gallagher and Andrew McKie

■ Introduction

Literature and poetry are being increasingly used as learning resources in professional health care educational curricula (McKie and Gass, 2001; Tschudin, 2003; McAteer and Murray, 2003; McKie et al., 2008). Less attention has, however, been given to specific ways in which engagement with these resources might enhance health care professionals' understanding of the experience of service users and carers and of their own practice with a view to improving health and social care practice.

In this chapter, we argue that literature and poetry have the potential to deepen professional understanding by literary devices such as metaphor, articulating, effectively, some of the most complex, elusive and subtle aspects of human experiences. Literature and poetry have the potential to enable professionals to develop ethical perception and imagination. The close attention that can be developed from reading poetry and literature is, arguably, transferable to practice contexts. Professionals can develop the ability to see more clearly the salient aspects of a practice situation. This is a precursor to ethical and professional practice. Poetry and literature are not the only resources that can be used to develop ethical perception or ethical practice. Insights from qualitative research and the visual arts are also valuable for enhancing ethical perception and ethical practice.

We begin with a general discussion of the relationship between the arts and health and social care offering some critique as well as a discussion of the benefits of the arts. We then discuss, more specifically, the potential of poetry and literature and consider claims that they enhance ethical perception. Metaphor is a common literary device and we consider its potential in relation to the experience of illness, distress and caring. In later sections we provide examples of literature and poetry in relation to the experience of service users, carers and professionals. We discuss practical ways in which the educationalist might adopt this approach in helping students and others to better understand and respond to the views and experiences of service users, carers and other professionals in different therapeutic and caring contexts.

■ Arts and humanities in health – The role of expression and criticality

The 'arts' represent an important component of culture and incorporate literature (including poetry), drawing, painting, sculpture, architecture and performing arts such as theatre music and dance. The arts are considered 'expressive' as they express, show or reveal something about the human condition. The humanities, on the other hand, as academic disciplines adopt a critical and analytical approach to the study of the human condition. Their broad scope is described as a 'bundle of disciplines' which includes theories of literature, music, art, history, theology and philosophy 'at the core' (Edgar and Pattison, 2006, p. 93). Recent additions to the humanities include religious, cultural, visual, postcolonial and feminist studies and, perhaps, social sciences such as sociology, anthropology and social psychology (ibid.). A concern over one main question unites these disciplines: 'What is it to be human?' Edgar and Pattison (2006, p. 93) put it this way:

> Within the humanities, this question – the question of how human beings understand, experience, and practise their own humanity – is typically addressed indirectly, by looking at the products of human existence, including language, beliefs, writings, paintings, and social institutions and organisations.

The relationship between the 'arts' and the health and social care professions can be characterised variously: as representing one component of professional practice (the 'art' as opposed to the 'science'); as providing creative resources to enhance people's understanding of the experience of receiving and giving care; and as activities that people can participate in creating their own visual, literary or performance work for recreational, therapeutic and educational purposes (Gallagher, 2007). But can anything count as a work of art? Carey (2005, p. 29), for example, argues that

> a work of art is anything that anyone has ever considered a work of art, though it may be a work of art only for that one person.

In addition, Ziff's (1997) question

> what is worthy of aesthetic appreciation?

is answered with the statement

anything that can be viewed.

It is of little consequence whether the extracts we draw on would receive the approval of an arts' critic. What matters is what the arts (particularly literature and poetry) express, how people engage with them and whether, and how, they make a difference to health and social care practice. Should we engage with the arts for their own sake or for some instrumental end? Are the arts useful or useless? Might they even be detrimental to health and social care practice, supporting a relativistic or subjective 'anything goes' stance? What might keep the arts on the ethical rails, so to speak?

■ The role of poetry and literature

In this chapter we are discussing the potential of poetry and literature in relation to health and social care. Understanding what we mean by these genres also determines our selection of material for later sections. Some definitions are more inclusive than others and, perhaps predictably, there is no consensus as to what can and should be included.

Poetry is derived from the Greek *poiesis*, which means 'making' or 'creating' and involves the use of language for aesthetic and expressive effect. It assumes many forms, ranging from concise Japanese haiku to epic poems, such as 'The Odyssey' and 'Kubla Khan'. Flanagan's view of poetry is as follows:

> the chiselled marble of language. It's a paint-spattered canvas – but the poet uses words instead of paint and the canvas is you.
>
> (http://contemporarylit.about.com/od/poetry/a/poetry.htm
> Accessed 20/11/07)

Flanagan further points out that one of the key features of poetry is its economy of language. He cites Wordsworth, who defined poetry as 'the spontaneous overflow of powerful feeling', and Dylan Thomas as saying, 'poetry is what makes me laugh or cry or yawn, what makes my toenails twinkle, what makes me want to do this or that or nothing'. Poetry uses many literary devices such as assonance, alliteration, rhythm, simile and metaphor. Conciseness of expression is a feature of some poetry and it has the potential to express, evoke and excite emotions. Poetry has the potential to convey meanings, feelings and perspectives.

Literature literally means 'acquaintance with letters' and is derived from the Latin *littera* meaning 'letter'. In its broadest sense, literature could include everything and anything that can be read: novels, plays, service user and professional narratives, professional case studies and reports. In a narrower sense, literature includes poetry, drama, essays, novels and short stories and often features plot, characters, storyline and, usually, has a clear beginning, middle and end. Literature might also be considered as material created by those acknowledged as authors or writers. We did not wish to restrict the scope of our definition of literature for our purposes. Some of the extracts of literature and poetry referred to in later sections were created by well-known authors and poets. Other extracts came from those with lived experience of health and social care.

The role of literature in illuminating a non-objective, constructed world of sensory, human experience cannot be overstated (Eagleton, 1983). Poetry, too – in its use of images, symbols and objects – can include, within its own multiple functions, an exploration of the diversity of human experience. It is the capacity of literature and poetry to translate these powers of description and imagination into 'mere words' that gives literature and poetry their potential to influence and transform human realities (Walker, 1997). According to Solzhenitsyn (1972), literature has the capacity to transcend human experience by distilling and offering that experience in new and accessible modes of human knowledge and understanding.

One of the claims made about literature is that it enhances the professional's ability to see or perceive. Pellegrino (1982), for example, writes of the relationship between medicine and literature:

> To look and to look feelingly is the summit of artistry for both medicine and literature; to take part in the struggle is the morality they share. Medicine and literature are linked, too, because both tell the story of what they see. The physician's history is really a tale, the narrative of a patient's odyssey in the dismal realms of disease, distress, disability and death. The writer, too, must contemplate the same perplexities of being human and being afflicted. Illness ever intrudes itself because it is inextricably woven and the tapestry of every human life.

It seems plausible that attention to stories or narratives may develop student professionals' ability to better perceive, or appreciate, the patient's perspective. This is also suggested by Montgomery Hunter et al. (1995):

> More specifically, literature has been included in the medical curriculum to develop students' narrative competencies, for example, the capacity to adopt others' perspectives, to follow the narrative thread of complex and chaotic stories, to tolerate ambiguity, and to recognise the multiple, often contradictory, meanings of events that befall human beings.

Downie (1991) suggests three ways in which the study of literature can be helpful. Firstly, literature can 'extend and give cognitive shaping to the sympathetic imagination'. Imaginative literature can develop empathy and enable doctors and nurses to perceive real need. Secondly, literature can help professionals come to terms with the emotions and conflicts which relate to those who are ill in a way philosophy or social sciences cannot. Thirdly, literature gives rise to moral questions which may challenge the self-perception of professionals.

There is, therefore, considerable optimism about what literature and, by association, poetry can achieve in relation to the professions. Assuming a sceptical stance is, however, important. Pickering (2000, p. 31) asks,

> when we do such-and-such, what are we doing? When we give health students a poem to read, what are we doing?

The arguments above suggest a range of benefits from engagement with literature; for example, the enhancement of perceptual and narrative capabilities, the ability to appreciate complexity and to tolerate ambiguity. But should we engage with the arts for their own sake or for such instrumental ends?

Pickering (2000, p. 31) argues that poetry has 'no instrumental use for purposes other than of trying to understand the poem in question'. Poetry should, therefore, be engaged with for its own sake, with a view to understanding and enjoying the poem rather than for the achievement of other ends:

> to read a poem as a resource is not to read it as a poem.

Reading a poem for 'external ends' is flawed because a poem is 'an event with necessarily unpredictable results'. Reading it for its own sake therefore acknowledges the significance of the poem–reader interaction and admits unpredictability of readers' responses. Any number of responses to, and interpretations of, a poem exist. Presenting a poem to students 'as a site where certain things have been found' precludes an invitation to students to read and engage with the poem for themselves (Pickering, 2000).

Responding to Pickering's claim that poetry is of no instrumental use, Ahlzen and Stolt (2001) argue that this unpredictability in terms of outcome and the possibility of multiple meanings is exactly what makes poetry valuable. Acknowledging the assumption within literary theory that meaning in a text is relational (residing 'neither in the text nor in the reader'), it is argued that engagement with poetry (reading, interpretation and discussion) *can* serve external or secondary ends. The usefulness of poetry and other literary texts in relation to medicine can be made

> because the clinical meeting is an encounter where the interpretation of words is crucial. Scientific explanations intersect with historical narrative in the clinical encounter. The clinical challenge par excellence is,

in our opinion, to be open to the patient's radical subjectivity, her ambiguity and complexity, and at the same time to apply the generalised, impersonal knowledge of scientific medicine. The clinician needs a language, and a mode of interpretation appropriate to both these aspects. Poetry reading can be a small but significant part of meeting this clinical challenge.

(Ahlen and Stolt, 2001, p. 48)

We are sympathetic to Pickering's argument that poetry should be read for its own sake. However, such reading necessarily gives rise to individual student interpretations that can be shared with others. The skills in sharing, comparing and contrasting interpretations could, arguably, be transferable to health and social care practice. Situations within health and social care give rise to many, sometimes conflicting, interpretations. We agree that the outcome of reading literature and poetry cannot, and should not, be predetermined and is unpredictable. The possibility that a student could interpret a text in a way that supports unethical practice should, at least, be considered. The possibility that a student could interpret a text in a way that devalues ethical practice should, at least, be considered. For example, Gunn's poem 'As Expected' (1982) might, for some readers, be interpreted as supporting seemingly more exciting career possibilities than working with people with learning disabilities. This poem will be discussed in a later section.

Could literature and poetry be detrimental to health and social care practice, supporting relativistic or subjective stances of 'anything goes'? It is certainly possible. The arts are expressive and encourage a range of different interpretations. It is the humanities that enable analysis and a critically reflective approach (Edgar and Pattison, 2006): engagement with philosophy (particularly moral philosophy) provides professionals with the means to describe and prescribe different ethical approaches to professional practice. The social sciences can provide evidence of the implications of practices that promote and thwart human flourishing (Waller, 1996). Exploring with students the *raison d'être* and values of their particular profession in relation to their reading of literature and poetry helps also to avoid relativism and subjectivism. By this, the arts can be kept on the ethical rails.

■ The meaning and significance of metaphor

Language has the potential to transform our understanding of the world via associative ways of comparison and contrast. The use of figural (pictorial) language, in contrast to literalness, points towards language's referential use (what it is 'about') rather than to its grammatical construction (what it 'says'). The associative power of language can be seen when we consider the use of simile and metaphor. Describing an experience can often be best achieved by comparing it to something else. Walker (1997) describes this as an association by analogy. Rush (2006) uses simile to describe the experience of loss following the death of his wife: 'I felt like a Pharaoh, the shell of a dead man.' Using the same device, Hicok (1988) describes a woman suffering from dementia:

She's like a fish in deep ocean, its body made of light.

The association between language and the ideas referred to in relation to metaphor is more complex. An example from Sontag (1991, edition) is illuminating:

Illness is the night-side of life, a more onerous citizenship. Everyone who is born holds dual citizenship, in the kingdom of the well and in the kingdom of the sick. Although we all prefer to use only the good passport, sooner or later each of us is obliged, at least for a spell, to identify ourselves as citizens of that other place.

Moving from one kingdom to another can be distressing, baffling, frightening or, perhaps, reassuring. Coming to terms with new contexts, conditions and expectations can be challenging and also rewarding for those who have travelled across kingdoms and for those who greet them, those who will travel with them until discharge or, in some instances, death.

Sontag's metaphor of dual citizenship is instructive and enlightening. Her discussion in relation to illnesses such as TB, cancer, insanity and AIDS details the range of perspectives conveyed by metaphor. Sontag's argument that illness is not a metaphor and that it is unhelpful to engage in 'metaphoric thinking' paradoxically, however, demonstrates its power and versatility to express societal values, political discourse and perspectives on the individual. Meaning in metaphor can change over time. Hanne and Hawken (2007), in a survey of illness metaphors in contemporary American media, note a 'softening' of the metaphors used to depict cancer and HIV/AIDS, alongside the use of more 'biomilitary' metaphors to describe other conditions: avian flu ('bioterrorist attack') and diabetes ('outwit the disease').

Metaphor can help, as does great art, to 'express the inexpressible' (Barker, 2000, p. 98). Considering illness as metaphor may have its limitations, but the power of metaphor to illuminate the experiences of illness remains persuasive. The term *metaphor* is derived from the Greek meaning 'transfer' or 'carry something across'. It has been described variously. Aristotle, for example, defined metaphor as 'the act of giving a thing a name that belongs to something else' (Aristotle, 1996, ed.: 34–35). More recently, Lakoff and Johnson (1980) demonstrated the pervasiveness of metaphor in everyday life by describing it as a means of 'understanding and experiencing one kind of thing in terms of another'. Several everyday metaphors could be used by service users: 'being at the end of my tether', 'unable to see the light at the end of tunnel', 'a shadow of their former selves' and 'so sharp you'll cut yourself' (Barker, 2000). Such commonplace use of metaphor can, however, be understood in deeper terms. By viewing hearing as a sensory experience prior to reading, metaphor can be understood as a device that moves away from literalness by seeking to draw the person *into* the reality of the issues under consideration (Paterson, 2006).

Hawkes (1972) writes of metaphor as involving a comparison or association between two objects or ideas with a view to bringing more clarity to bear:

> The effect of metaphor 'properly' used is that by combining the familiar with the unfamiliar, it adds charm and distinction, to clarity. Clarity comes from 'everyday words', the 'proper or regular class' of terms used by everybody in conversation. Charm comes from the intellectual pleasure afforded by the new resemblances noted in the metaphor, distinction from the surprising nature of some of the resemblances discerned.
>
> (Hawkes, 1972, p. 9)

The use of everyday words and ideas to illuminate or clarify is evident in the metaphors within the extracts that follow. In the first, Elie Wiesal's account of his boyhood experiences in the Buchenwald concentration camp during the Second World War richly uses metaphor for descriptive and meaning-creating purposes (Wiesal, 1960). The following excerpt captures something of this influence:

> Not far from us there were some prisoners at work. Some were digging holes, others carrying sand. None of them so much as glanced at us. We were so many dried-up trees in the heart of a desert. Behind me, some people were talking. I had not the slightest desire to listen to what they were saying, to know who was talking or what they were talking about. No one dared to raise his voice, though there was no supervisor near us. Perhaps it was because of the thick smoke which poisoned the air and took one by the throat [...].

Wiesal's description of the camp experience in terms of 'so many dried-up trees in the heart of a desert' is one metaphorical way of conveying something of the prisoners' collective experience. In literal terms, human beings are not trees. However, the use of the image of 'dried-up trees' – suggestive of experience marked by parchedness, thirst, heat, exhaustion and dispiritedness – enhances the potential for the reader to understand the terrible conditions experienced by the author. Moreover, the influence of this particular metaphor is further sharpened by locating it within the narrative preceding it. Here, the account of other prisoners labouring (digging holes and moving sand) adds to the power of Wiesal's metaphor. Similarly, the use of the metaphor 'poisoned' to describe the smoke in the camp suggests a wider and deeper atmosphere whose all-pervasive effect is to choke and stifle communication amongst the prisoners, even when their guards are not physically present.

A second example comes from a poem entitled 'Old Woman', written by Kenneth Stevens (2000).

> [...] Once she was beautiful, and knew it;
> Once her blood's fire burned in a man's veins
> Night after night, and her colours
> Enflamed the coals of his heart.
>
> Who may see that now,
> When the nurses bring her things and swear
> Behind her back because she cannot hold
> A spoon, or manage all the stairs?
>
> (2000)

Stevens uses metaphor to illustrate several dimensions of the human experience of ageing. By using the metaphors of 'fire' and 'coals' to describe the woman's present state and how she once affected others, the poem challenges readers to consider the women and, perhaps, older people they work with in ways characterised by the depth of understanding and recognition of personhood and the narrative and dignity of a life.

Engagement with literature and poetry in relation to practitioners' personal and professional practice requires careful and sensitive facilitation on the part of educators. The discussion of Stevens' poem took place within the context of a poetry workshop organised by one of us (A.McK.). Stevens, a Scottish poet, led this workshop, where nursing students were requested to read in advance a poetry sourcebook containing five of Stevens' own published poems. Meeting the author in such settings can potentially help practitioners overcome deeply rooted obstacles to engaging with literary sources. Careful facilitation of such sessions – for example, sketching in the background to a particular poem or excerpt (Stevens was for a time employed as a cleaner in a nursing home) – can do much to enhance practitioners' learning experience.

Two further points deserve consideration. Firstly, although the act of reading may often appear in individualised and 'privatised' terms, innovative forms of learning within communal settings (e.g. reading 'aloud' or in triads) can counter charges of 'ethical relativism' and subjectivism (Slagter, 2007). Secondly, by encouraging practitioners to identify their own choices of literature and poetry and to bring these into discussion of ethical practice alongside current professional approaches to ethics, notions of a predetermined and 'acceptable' canon of sources chosen by educationalists can be disavowed (Begley, 2003).

In summary, the impact of metaphor as used in literature and poetry lies in its ability to draw the reader into a wider framework of reference. Metaphor creates new understanding through difference and can be seen as a microscopic representation of a larger body of work (Ricoeur, 1991). Metaphor, in its ability to nurture insight via difference or even ambiguity, is presented as a powerful way of understanding. It is also an engaging way to assist understanding. In addition to reading poetry, professionals and service users may write their own poetry. For service users, the power of writing as a therapeutic tool to promote self-understanding and healing has for some time been recognised (Bolton, 1999; McAndle and Bynt, 2001). In different, but related ways also, it can help professionals understand better the experience of service users and their own experience as professionals.

In the next section we include extracts from Gunn's poem and extracts from literature. Given the wealth of material, this selection was challenging. Our selection rationale was threefold: the extracts illustrate the role of metaphor and simile; they have the potential to facilitate rich and diverse interpretations; and they reveal the experiences and perspectives of the service user, carer and professionals.

■ The potential of poetry and literature

A wide range and variety of poetry is worthy of exploration and might have been included in this section. One of us (AMcK) co-facilitates an Expressive Arts module, which has collated four poetry sourcebooks. Mindful of Pickering's critique, we invite you, as readers, to consider different interpretations and how these might contribute to, or detract from, professional practice. Below are extracts from Gunn's poem 'As expected' (1982). We strongly recommend that you access the poem in its entirety in Gunn (1982). Read the poem aloud and consider what it makes you feel and think and, if possible, compare your reading and interpretation with that of others.

> *As Expected*
>
> *Most of his friends, as expected,*
> *went into service. Two*
> *became pilots,[......].*
>
> *Larry chose a slower route.*
>
> *He was assigned a grubby*
> *roomful of young men sitting around*
> *idle, or idle on their cots[......]*

They looked like ninepins
But he found that none had head-lice
and let them grow their hair.
They started to look as if they had different names[. . . .]

Larry watched: if the unteachable
can teach themselves, it follows
they can be taught by others.

One learned to eat without help [. . . . . . .]

[. . . . .] stumbling like kittens, inarticulate
like tulips bending in a west wind,
and learning as they went, like humans.

(Gunn, 1982)

We recognise that many practitioners may find discussion of this poem challenging. It may be possible, however, to facilitate such discussion via several approaches. Here are a few:

- *The use of simile and metaphor in fostering new understanding via difference. For example*:

  What images of the young men are conveyed by describing them as 'like ninepins'?
  In what ways can learning be compared to stumbling 'like kittens' and 'inarticulate like tulips'?
  What understanding might be gained about Larry as a person in his choice of a 'slower route' for a possible career?

- *Discussion of relevant themes.* For example,

  After reading the poem in its entirety, in what ways can you identify with Gunn's account in the first three stanzas of the issues involved in deciding upon a career devoted to helping others?
  Is it possible to see every person as unique?
  What might be understood by the young men having 'different names'?

- *Moments of insight.* For example:

  Again when reading the poem as a whole, what moments of insight for Larry can you identify?
  In what ways can you relate these to your own learning experiences in practice?

The next three extracts of literature are in prose rather than poetic form. Two are from Padfield's book *Perceptions of Pain* (2003). The book focuses on the experience of pain and on photographic representations of pain. Although the focus of the book is on visualisation, the written accounts from those who experience pain are very graphic and utilise a range of metaphors:

> I describe it as a cement mixer because of the density of wet cement. It feels like cement being poured down my throat and filling up my body and I can't stop it. For other people with breathing difficulties, they might see it as water filling them up, but for me it is something heavy weighing down on my chest so that I cannot move.
>
> (Dwoskin, 2003, p. 108)

and

> I see a huge rubbish tip that has mounds of rubbish in it. It feels to me that there comes a point in my pain where I feel that things are under control and running along fairly smoothly, when suddenly another load of rubbish is poured onto the site and I am back to square one. It can be other people's rubbish, it can be change of medication, it can be anything. I can never be truly in control or get the rubbish level and smooth, because always something comes along and makes it mountainous again. It is absolute chaos and the feeling that people come along once a day or a week and just dump more rubbish on the tip.
>
> (Brooks, 2003, p. 86)

The final extract is from a mother's perspective. She describes her experience of waiting for her 14-year-old daughter to undergo surgery:

> Lindsay in the side-ward lay greenly gowned with her hair drawn up in a complex plait from crown to nape. I waded to her against the drag of a fierce ebb-tide, walking against time to where she would soon not be. In the crook of one slender bare arm, rosy with eczema, lay her toy cat disinterred from the childhood she had sought to put behind her.
>   'The nurse did the plait for me. I've got to have my bowels done.'
>   'I know.'
>   'Don't cry.'
>   'I'm not.'
>   The child in me was weeping scalding storms; but my daughter and I remained dry-eyed. She neither clung not offered a token of fear. Her bravery stabbed me with pangs of an obscure remorse.
>
> (Davies, 2002, p. 36)

These extracts reveal a range of perspectives on institutionalisation, pain and remorse. 'As Expected' invites rich and diverse interpretations and reveals something of the experience of a young man working in an institution. The poem was the focus of Pickering's discussion regarding the uselessness of poetry. It is important to note also the historical context of the poem. Readers have the benefit, perhaps ironically, of consulting and comparing their interpretation of the poem with his (Pickering, 2000).

The extracts from Dwoskin and Brooks, utilising metaphor and simile, graphically illustrate the burden of breathing difficulties and pain in terms of 'wet cement' filling up a body, as unstoppable and as 'more rubbish on the tip'. The Davies example expresses the challenges experienced by a parent when her teenage daughter undergoes surgery and her difficulty in getting close ('against the drag of a fierce ebb-tide') and of regression and sadness perhaps ('the child in me was weeping scalding storms'). Readers may well focus on different aspects of these extracts and have different interpretations as to what is expressed.

■ Practical hints and challenges

Some of these have already been discussed in considering Stevens' poem 'Old Woman' (Stevens, 2000) and Gunn's 'As Expected' (Gunn, 1982). Other features may, however, be helpful for educationalists considering the use of literature and poetry in professional health and social care settings:

- To make the link between reading and practice clearer, requesting practitioners to write a short (400–500 words) essay by way of their response to a particular poem or literary extract. This can be discussed in workshop format, but it can also be used formatively to help practitioners make connections between reading literary sources and their own personal and professional experience (Sakalys, 2002).
- Employing a range of reading sources (e.g. 'classics', 'popular' titles, users' and carers' work) to suit the possible range of practitioners' reading habits, professional experience and personal interests.
- Run workshops or discussion forums in structured, but informal and friendly, ways; for example, incorporating refreshment breaks.
- Careful consideration of timing within the curricula in introducing practitioners to literary sources (Macnaughton, 2000; Smith et al. 2006).
- On the part of educationalists, fostering patience and sensitivity to where practitioners are, but being prepared for the unexpected and the surprising.

To promote reflection using metaphors, in relation to specific poems, literature and practice experiences, educationalists might invite students to do the following tasks:

- Consider a poem or novel that you have read recently. Try to link your responses to it with aspects of your own current practice.

- Think of three metaphors that could be used to describe your own recent practice.
- Note ways in which these metaphors might help in understanding your practice better.

■ Conclusion

The experiences of people who avail themselves of, and deliver, health and social care services are unique, unusual, common and applicable to all. Scott (2000, p. 5) cites from Gordon Allport as follows:

> each person is like every other person, like some other people, like no other person. Each of us contains within us both general patterns and the particular, that which is peculiar to me and my context.

This chapter has sought to show how literature and poetry can be used in the educational preparation of professional health carers. By identifying the expressive and critical role of the arts and humanities in health care, these sources can serve as relevant means of helping health care professionals to better understand the world of patients, clients, practice and care settings. The power of metaphor is offered as one means of facilitating this learning by ways of understanding experience by highlighting and exploring difference and similarity. This potential to transform understanding of clients' experience is demonstrated through consideration of several prose and poetry examples. No guarantee can be given that practice change will occur as a result of such engagement. Nevertheless, we invite educational programme leaders to consider the spirit of Allport's observation in relation to the rich potential that engagement with literature and poetry can offer to professional health care education today.

References

Ahlzen, R. and Stolt, C.-M. (2001) Poetry, interpretation and unpredictability: A reply to Neil Pickering. *Journal of Medical Ethics: Medical Humanities*. 27, 47–49.

Aristotle (1996) *Poetics*. Heath, M. (trans.) Penguin, London.

Barker, P. (2000) Working with the metaphor of life and death. *Journal of Medical Ethics: Medical Humanities*. 26, 97–102.

Begley, A.-M. (2003) Creative approaches to ethics: Poetry, prose and dialogue. In Tschudin, V. (ed.) *Approaches to Ethics – Nursing Beyond Boundaries*. Butterworth-Heinemann, London.

Bolton, G. (1999) *The Therapeutic Potential of Creative Writing. Writing Myself*. Jessica Kingsley Publishers Ltd., London.

Brooks, R. (2003) I have been asked to describe my pain.... In Padfield, D. (ed.) *Perceptions of Pain*. Dewi Lewis Publishing, Stockport, p. 86.

Carey, J. (2005) *What Good Are the Arts?* Faber & Faber, London.

Davies, S. (2002) Inside Out. In Morley, D. (ed.) *The Gift: New Writing for the NHS.* Stride Publications, Devon.

Downie, R. (1991) Literature and Medicine. *Journal of Medical Ethics.* 17, 93–98.

Dwoskin, S. (2003) I describe it as a cement mixer.... In Padfield, D. (ed.) *Perceptions of Pain.* Dewi Lewis Publishing, Stockport, p. 86.

Eagleton, T. (1983) *Literary Theory – An Introduction.* Blackwell Pub. Ltd., Oxford.

Edgar, A. and Pattison, S. (2006) Need the humanities be so useless? Justifying the place and role of the humanities as a critical resource for performance and practice. *Journal of Medical Ethics: Medical Humanities.* 32, 2, 92–98.

Gallagher, A. (2007) The role of the arts in mental health nursing: Emperor's new suit or magic pill? *Journal of Psychiatric and Mental Health Nursing.* 14, 424–429.

Gunn, G. (1982) *The Passages of Joy.* Faber and Faber, London.

Hanne, M. and Hawken, S. J. (2007) Metaphors for illness in contemporary media. *Journal of Medical Ethics: Medical Humanities.* 33, 2, 93–99.

Hawkes, E. (1972) *Metaphor.* Metheun Co. Ltd., London.

Hicok, R. (1988) Alzheimer's. In Astley, N. (ed.) (2004) *Being Alive.* Bloodaxe Books, Northumberland.

Lakoff, G. and Johnson, M. (1980) *Metaphors We Live By.* University of Chicago Press, Chicago/London.

Macnaughton, J. (2000) The humanities in medical education: Context, outcomes and structures. *Journal of Medical Ethics: Medical Humanities.* 26, 23–30.

McAndle, S. and Bynt, R. (2001) Fiction, poetry and mental health: Expressive and therapeutic uses of literature. *Journal of Psychiatric and Mental Health Nursing.* 8, 517–524.

McAteer, M. and Murray, R. (2003) The humanities in a course on loss and grief. *Physiotherapy.* 89, 2, 97–103.

McKie, A. and Gass, J. P. (2001) Understanding mental health through reading selected literature sources: An evaluation. *Nurse Education Today.* 21, 3, 201–208.

McKie, A., Adams, V., Gass, J. P. and Macduff, C. (2008) Windows and mirrors: Reflections of a module team teaching the arts in nurse education. *Nurse Education in Practice.* 8, 156–164.

Montgomery Hunter, K., Charon, R. and Coulehan, J. L. (1995) The study of literature in medical education. *Academic Medicine.* 70, 9, 787–791.

Paterson, E. (2006) *Eat this Book – The Art of Spiritual Reading.* Hodder & Stoughton, London.

Pellegrino, E. D. (1982) To look feelingly – The affinities of medicine and literature. *Literature and Medicine.* 1, 18–22.

Pickering, N. (2000) The use of poetry in health care ethics education. *Journal of Medical Ethics: Medical Humanities.* 26, 31–36.

Ricoeur, P. (1991). *From Text to Action: Essays in Hermeneutics II* (translated by Kathleen Blamey and John B), Northwestern University Press, Thompson, U.S.

Rush, C. (2006) *To Travel Hopefully Journal of a Death not Foretold.* Profile Books, London.

Sakalys, J. A. (2002) Literary pedagogy in nursing: A theory-based perspective. *Journal of Nursing Education.* 41, 9, 386–392.

Scott, P. A. (2000) The relationship between the arts and medicine. *Journal of Medical Ethics: Medical Humanities.* 26, 1, 3–8.

Slagter, C. G. (2007) Approaching interpretive virtues through reading aloud. In Smith, D. I., Shortt, J. and Sullivan, J. (eds.) *Teaching Spiritually Engaged Reading.* The Stapleford Centre, Nottingham.

Smith, S., Molineux, M., Rowe, N. and Larkinson, L. (2006) Integrating medical humanities in physiotherapy and occupational therapy education. *International Journal of Therapy and Rehabilitation.* 13, 9, 421–427.

Solzhenitsyn, A. (1972) *The Nobel Prize Lecture.* Stenvalley Press, London.

Sontag, S. (1991) *Illness as Metaphor.* Penguin Books, UK.

Stevens, K. (2000) Old Woman from *Iona.* Saint Andrews Press, Edinburgh.

Tschudin, V. (2003) (ed.) *Approaches to Ethics – Nursing Beyond Boundaries.* Butterworth-Heinemann, London.

Walker, C. A. (1997) Imagination, metaphor and nursing theory. *Journal of Theory Construction and Testing.* 1, 1, 22–27.

Waller, J. E. (1996) Perpetrators of the Holocaust: Divided and unitary self conceptions of evildoing. *Holocaust and Genocide Studies.* 10, 1, 11–33.

Wiesal, E. (1960) *Night.* Avon Books, New York.

Ziff, P. (1997) Anything viewed. In Feagin, S. and Maynard, P. (eds) *Aesthetics.* Oxford University Press, pp. 23–30.

Chapter 9

Portraying an abstract landscape: Using painting to develop self-awareness and sensitive practice

Sue McAndrew and Tony Warne

■ Introduction

Contemporary health and social care practice promotes the notion of developing an emotionally intelligent practitioner and, in wanting such, recognises the impact of self-awareness and reflexive practice on the quality of patient experience. Developing a heightened level of self-awareness is a continual requirement for professional practice. It is contended that a practitioner's self-examination is crucial to patient's progress, as it facilitates the recognition of how their own issues may impact on their reception and understanding of what the patient presents with (Goldberg, 1993). This chapter looks at the way such reflective learning can be facilitated through the use of art; that is, painting experience. Effectively facilitated, reflective learning on practice through use of art will stimulate self-awareness and personal growth, thus enhancing the health and social care professionals' practice. The chapter draws upon work undertaken by us with groups of student nurses, at different stages of their training, who using paints, were given opportunity to reflect on their experience and make sense of their emotional self in relation to some of the people they encountered in clinical practice.

■ A portrait of self

Arguably, the ability to manage our own emotional life whilst attending to and interpreting other people's is a prerequisite skill for any caring profession. Reluctance on the part of the practitioner to work with the emotionality often inherent in interpersonal relationships could be the result of their own internal psyche, influenced by their own social, cultural and political identity. Such experiences will have a direct impact on their openness and willingness to explore intimate and sensitive issues with others. Health and social care practice is often experienced as being emotionally charged and will elicit different emotional responses in different professionals. One explanation for this might be the individual's unconscious processes that trigger an emotional response to a particular situation, person or issue. However, such emotional response may be experienced as an anathema to the professional persona, thus creating feelings of confusion and insecurity. If or when this occurs, health and social care professionals are more likely to feel insecure in addressing emotional, intimate and/or sensitive issues and, as a consequence, might try to assert competence and control through use of defence mechanisms. Professional detachment, splitting, denial of personal feelings, the use of rhetoric and the pathologising of what we do not understand are all defence mechanisms commonly adopted by health professionals (Warne and McAndrew, 2005a). In particular, splitting is often used as a defence mechanism to suspend emotional distress in order to engage in our work life; for example, the nurse having awareness that the patient is experiencing mental pain, but convincing herself that she is only there to deal with physical health problems. This would enable the nurse to carry out a nursing task without getting caught up in the maelstrom of emotion inherent in the interpersonal interaction with the patient. In this way splitting as a defence mechanism acts as an unconscious coping strategy that allows the nurse to deal with the emotional labour of caring.

Whilst we would not advocate stripping away a student's defence mechanisms, bringing some to conscious awareness offers the student the opportunity to make more informed choices regarding the way in which they practice. In gaining insight and a better understanding of their own unconscious defences, practitioners will be more adept in avoiding the generation and perpetuation of negative feelings and poor treatment decisions (Warne and McAndrew, 2005b). In relinquishing some of their defence mechanisms, health and social care professionals will be free to learn new ways of viewing and dealing with the world.

For example, in one of the reflective sessions, one of the students painted a picture depicting herself and a lady she was caring for, who after 50 years of marriage was bereaved following the death of her husband. Between herself and the lady, the student had painted a tree. The student's explanation for the tree was that it depicted bringing new life to the lady and represented the student's efforts in encouraging the lady to participate in social activity groups within a day care setting. The lady refused to engage and the student felt helpless. When exploring the painting, it became obvious to the student that whilst the tree provided a 'safe' space between herself and the patient it also formed a barrier between them. At a conscious level, one interpretation would be that the student was trying to 'mend' the patient's life by presenting her with activities that would distract her from her sadness. At an unconscious level, a different interpretation might be that the student found the lady's emotional state too painful to bear and what the tree represented was the splitting of the lady's sadness from the student's need to make her life happy, professional detachment and/or the denial of her own emotional response to the lady's pain.

These conscious and unconscious strategies form part of the emotional labour of caring (Hochschild, 1983; Mann, 2006). In trying to engage the patient in activities the student is hoping to put an end to the patient's emotional distress and thus unconsciously contain her own distress. However, paradoxically, in doing this, the student adds to her own distress, which is then consciously experienced as helplessness.

There is a further paradox revealed in this example. Whilst, as educationalists, the painting and subsequent deconstruction of the student's experience presents a useful learning opportunity, it is one which is also risky in terms of the student's psyche and sense of self in relation to simultaneously being a novice practitioner, a student and a human being. Thus, as educationalists, we need to consider how the novice practitioner can capture the essence of the interpersonal relationship in a constructive way that harnesses their naivety in order to translate their learning into personal and interpersonal knowing.

■ Making sense of the abstract: The art of nursing

As educationalists, it is the process of sense-making that should lie at the core of the student's learning. Teachers have the opportunity to make connections with the historical traditions that provide them and their students with a voice, history and a sense of belonging (Searle, 1992). However, it has been suggested (Warne and McAndrew, 2006) that just as nurses avoid addressing emotional issues with their patients, those delivering the curriculum can avoid teaching emotionality by becoming 'lost' in the milieu of higher education. Again this could be defensive on the part of educators. Like the students they are teaching, they will have their own internal psyche, shaped by their own social, cultural and political identity influencing their educative practices. For some, the familiar educational processes inherent in higher education provide a sense of ontological security in dealing with the turbulence of emotionality. Indeed, in a culture that values academic achievement, emotional aspects of caring become more marginalised (Gilmartin, 2000). The result is that the student can become discouraged from questioning their teachers and, as they move towards qualified practitioner, lose all motivation to resist the confining habitus of professional practice (Scott, 2003).

As stated in the introductory chapter, if the aim of contemporary health and social care education is to create reflective, emotionally intelligent practitioners, correct educational processes and support systems are put in place so that students are able to flourish (Nolan et al., 1995). In order to achieve this some educators will need to broaden and develop their own teaching practices if the rhetoric of the emotionally intelligent practitioner is to come to fruition. Teachers who are sensitive to their students and who themselves are emotionally expressive are likely to encourage exploration (Rogers, 1993). In aspiring to achieve the emotionally intelligent practitioner, educators need to learn how to better listen to the students they work with in order to find out what it is they know and understand about the lives of the people they are working with in practice. In doing so they will begin to learn what it is the student wants to achieve and what help is required in order to meet their learning needs. In this scenario the student experience becomes the centre of their educational universe. To expedite this requires creating the opportunity for personalising the educational process through validating the emotional context of the student's personal experiences as the foundation for their learning. There has to be a willingness to engage with and be engaged in, the ability to momentarily stop the internal didactic teacher, in pursuit of reflectively searching for the meanings constructed within the interpersonal encounter.

The process for creating such opportunities has to be more than simply encouraging the student to tell their story. As we have seen in Chapter 3, stories are a useful medium for learning about the lives and problems of others. In using paint as a medium for storytelling the dynamic of emotion can be easily introduced into the process by using colour to represent the emotions specific to a particular interpersonal encounter. The teacher is required to listen to and understand the ways in which the student makes sense of their feelings or the feelings they have when they are with patients. This will be achieved by asking probing and challenging questions so that possibilities of transference and counter-transference are recognised and used as possible learning opportunities. The teacher can then verify these understandings. Through interactive dialogue with the student and the rest of their peer group, acting as a catalyst for translating the expressed experience into learning possibilities, the emotional context of their experience will be enhanced. Thus in making such connections with the student and their personal clinical experience the important component of emotionality will become integral to the educational process.

■ Colouring the landscape: Using art in reflective education

In using art as a reflective tool, it is the unconscious primary process of knowing 'self' and the impact of that 'self' in the interpersonal relationship that we are trying to elicit in the student. In moving towards the emotionally intelligent practitioner it is the 'emotional' component of the inter-subjective relationship that needs to be captured, through symbolic representation of the affective experience. One way of achieving this is through symbolic expression used in painting. The flow of the paint, the symbolic representation of the picture and the colour all promote a safe space to get in touch with feelings in their most vivid form (Bateman and Holmes, 1995).

■   Framing a safe space

To facilitate any teaching session, where integral to the session is the exploration of emotions, is risky and needs careful preparation. At a pragmatic level part of preparing the safe environment will require the establishment of functional boundaries; for example, the timings of the session, how the session will be organised, and clear instructions with regard to the expectations we have of the students as individuals and as a group.

For most of the groups that we have worked with painting is something that most of the students have not encountered since their schooldays. By giving recognition to this fact and reassuring the students that we are not looking for 'Van Goughs' the process of putting people at ease can start. The group are asked to paint a particular topic; for example, someone they have worked with who has experienced low self-esteem, loss or difficulty accepting their illness. To continue the process of putting the students at ease, when explaining what we want the students to do, we suggest that they can paint the picture in any form of their choice; for example, a picture, symbols, matchstick, people and so on. Emphasis is given to the fact that as long as the painting has meaning for the student and they can explain their painting to the group, how they chose to paint the scenario will be acceptable. A similar explanation is given to the use of colour. In this instance we suggest that the student think about and use colour to represent the emotions of the moment the picture captures, but that we, as educationalists, 'read' nothing into the use of a particular colour; so if for one student red represents happiness then so be it.

As with any experiential learning, reluctant students might need a more one-to-one encounter in order to help them get started. Reiterating the process and affirming that the student has control over what they paint and what they chose to share with the group can help allay some fears. In engaging in a reflective process such as this, for educationalists the bottom line is that of protecting the students from harm. With this in mind we would recommend that if using painting to reflect on practice the session be facilitated by two teachers, one of whom can be readily available if any of the students become distressed during the process whilst the other can continue with the group. Lastly, before letting them get started with their painting, we ask them, as adults, to 'just give it a go and let's see where it takes us'. Our practice is then to give psychological space by, once they all have got started, physically leaving the room so they can get on with their painting without feeling inhibited by our presence.

■ Loading the brush

In providing an insight into how we have used painting we will use the example of addressing the concept of loss. The students are asked to think about a patient they have looked after in clinical practice who has experienced a loss. This involves loss in its broadest sense: physical loss, a limb, mobility, breast; and/or emotional loss, a relationship, self-esteem, confidence. The student is then asked to paint a picture representing the patient and their loss, using colour to capture the patient's mood. Once the student has completed this part of the picture, they are then asked to paint themselves into the picture.

■ Colouring me

Asking the student to situate their self in relation to this experience provides an opportunity for the student to safely deconstruct their experiences in terms of conceptual and experiential ways of knowing. When asked to paint themselves into the painting they are asked to think about the use of colour to reflect their own feelings when they are with the patient in their picture. In addition, before painting themselves into the picture they have to think about proximity with regard to how close they feel to the patient and how large or small they need to paint themselves in relation to how much involvement they think they have in the patient's life.

■ Examples from practice

We use two examples here to illustrate the kind of paintings produced by students and a brief synopsis of the classroom discussion that is used as a prompt for group learning and direction towards theoretical connections. The paintings and the student accounts belong to the students. Permission to use these in this chapter has been given by the students involved.

☐ Example one

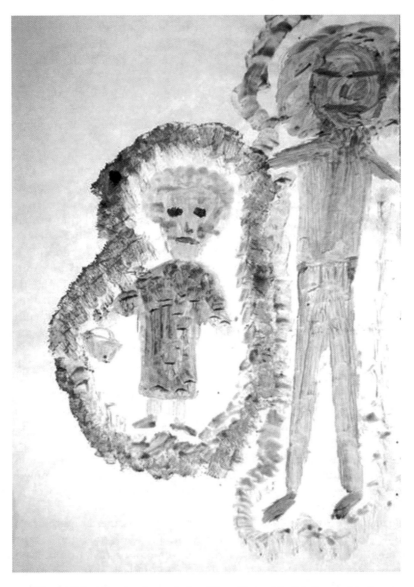

Figure 9.1 Blurring boundaries: The widow who didn't wear black.

Figure 9.1 shows a 58-year-old lady who has recently been widowed. She is tall and slim and 'does not look her age'. She has been referred for depression but describes herself as 'lost'. Whilst the grief resulting from her husband's death, painted as a black wavy blurred line encompassing the lady, acts as a blurred boundary surrounding her and at the same time it 'cocoons' her. The student has painted herself as smaller than the lady but, like her, the student is also encompassed by a blue wavy line albeit a much stronger line than the one surrounding the patient. Whilst the line encompassing the student is blue, the student has painted her own body in black. Both the student and the patient share the same colours.

When the student starts telling the story of her painting she tells the group that 'her patient is a stereotypical widow but she never wears black'. The student is irritated by this and questions what help this lady needs given that 'she seems to be managing ok'. Picking up on her statements, we discuss incongruence when expected behaviour does not match with what is being presented. Some of the student's colleagues ask why both herself and the patient are 'boxed in'. After considering her response to this question, and on closer exploration of her own painting, the student suggests that just as the patient is completely surrounded by her grief over her husband's death, she feels overwhelmed by the lady's grief and this restricts her ability to help the lady. The student states that she also feels 'lost' and helpless. The notions of 'stereotypical widow', 'helplessness' and 'lost' are captured and written on the whiteboard and when the student has completed her story we return to them and consider what theories each might link to. With regard to the former we consider theories of labelling and cultural and social expectations. In terms of helplessness we identified Seligman's concepts of helplessness and hopelessness, and with regard to feeling lost, Worden and Kublar-Ross's theories of grief, in particular that of searching for that which is lost, are considered.

When exploring the emotional aspects of self inherent in the picture the student focused on the line surrounding her and what it was about her that had prompted the painting of self in this way. The picture depicts that of the student nurse wearing black and being cocooned. The student talked of the patient frustrating her and after unpacking her frustration she thought that the basis of such feelings lay in the patient's failure to comply with accepted social norms – 'widows wear black; otherwise they can't be really grieving – can they?' The student then said that she 'would wear black' and indeed painted herself doing so in the picture. As mentioned above, we briefly explored the cultural and social influences on these ideas, but this then led the group to engage in a discussion about social attitudes, values and beliefs and how these 'fitted' the Rogerian concept of unconditional positive regard. As a group the students recognised that as human beings we do bring something of our self to the interpersonal encounter and how important it is to develop strategies – for example clinical supervision – to help us differentiate what belongs to the patient and what belongs to us and to ensure our own attitudes, value and beliefs do not hinder and/or compromise the relationship.

☐   Example two

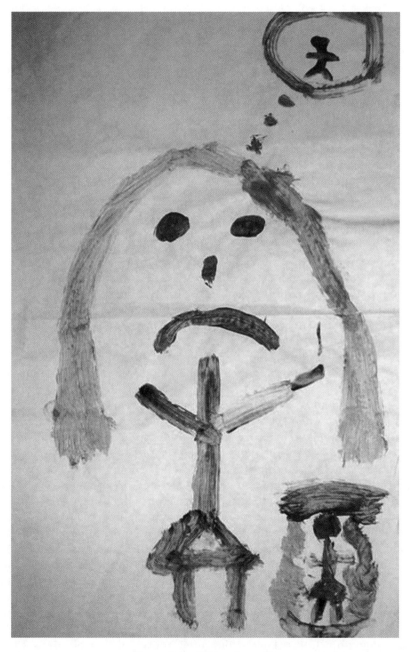

Figure 9.2   Filling the void.

Figure 9.2 shows Jane, a 39-year-old lady whose only child was taken into care 18 years ago after her partner at that time was convicted of paedophilia. Jane had recently been in touch with her daughter in the hope of re-establishing the relationship. However, things had not worked out and her daughter had refused to have any further contact with her, leaving Jane frustrated and depressed.

Jane occupies the main space in the painting, with thoughts of her daughter being in a bubble at the top right-hand corner of the picture. At times Jane is angry with her daughter for refusing to try and re-establish their relationship but at other times she is sad (painted in green to depict the sadness) and longs for the 'lost relationship'. Jane describes her life to the student as 'empty', her body being bereft of her child. The student has worked closely with Jane, engaging her in activities such as going out shopping and visiting Jane at her flat to help her sort out some things that she wanted to do. The student describes Jane as 'a very kind lady', who is always asking her how her university work is going and what she has been doing during the weekend and shows a general interest in her well-being. In the painting the student appears in the lower right-hand corner and paints herself in three of the four colours she has used to paint Jane in. Additionally, the student has some red around her linking her to Jane's thoughts about her own daughter. The student feels she has made good progress with Jane but wishes 'more than anything' that 'her daughter would re-contact her and have another go at trying to make the relationship work'. The student sees Jane as 'someone who would be a really good mother given the chance'.

When conveying her story the student started to realise what might be happening in her own relationship with Jane. The student is of similar age as Jane's daughter and when Jane asks her about her personal life the student readily shares information with Jane. When retelling Jane's story to the group the student began to realise that when with Jane she herself acted in a similar way to when she was with her own mother. The student, on her return home, would tell her mother what she had been doing at university, where she had been with friends and so on, and she now spoke to Jane about the same sorts of things. Whilst this realisation was somewhat alarming for the student we did explore surrogacy and re-enactment as positive attributes in working therapeutically with patients. In raising these concepts the work of Peplau and using a psychodynamic approach to therapy were considered. A couple of other students brought up the notion of 'parent–child' communication within the framework of transactional analysis and the student telling the story found this useful in terms of sense-making and also in thinking about how she might change the present scenario. With regard to the latter, Egan's work *The Skilled Helper* was then considered.

At an emotional level the student quickly became aware that she and Jane were painted in the same colours, indicating that they shared the same emotions. Just as Jane at times felt angry with herself, the student felt angry with Jane's daughter. Likewise, when Jane was sad the student felt sad and it was at these times that the student was more likely to share parts of 'self' with Jane. Again we explored the similarities between her own and Jane's feelings and how certain feelings elicited certain responses. During this dialogue the student was also able to consider why she made the assumption that Jane was someone who would make a really good mother and what she (the student) actually meant by this. In bringing these issues to the fore within the group we were able to discuss transference, counter-transference, intuition, attachment theory and Winnicott's work relating to the 'good enough mother'.

☐ Completing the picture

Throughout the session, and as mentioned in Example 1, as each student tells the story of their painting, re-occurring themes are captured and recorded on the whiteboard. Once all the students have told their stories and unpacked their paintings, as a group we look at the themes that have emerged and think about which theoretical concepts would link to and help make sense of a particular theme. Whilst some of the themes that emerge are easily accessible in terms of the students being able to link them to theory they have previously learnt, others might link to theories they are less familiar with. In the case of the latter, a short reading list that is linked to particular themes can later be given to the students.

Asking adults to paint is often experienced as a threatening activity and counter-intuitive to the understanding of traditional adult education. As you can see from the pictures, asking someone to paint unconsciously takes them back to childhood, but in our experience to what Berne (1961) described as the 'free child', where the emotional self becomes transparent. In doing so, multiple layers of resonance and meaning are evoked by symbolic representation and colour (Mann, 2006). The pictures that the students produce allow us, as educationalists, to explore the multiple layers of the interpersonal relationship, with different aspects of health and social care practices becoming apparent at different times.

Whilst at a superficial level this might appear a simple process, the reality is that of a very sensitive complex process. On the part of the student it is not merely telling the story through the picture, but an often-cathartic experience that has to be held and contained. On the part of the educationalist the process requires utilisation of very complex skills that involve asking questions that would invite elaboration on recent practice, whilst at the same time ensuring a safe environment for exploration. Again we return to the notion of safety, and in this instance it is important not to make judgements on the quality of the pictures as this may cloud the experience as one of negativity and will close down imagination. We would advocate that what is important is the validating of the student's interpretation of the symbolism, picture and colour as a vehicle for learning.

■ Sharing, caring and learning

As suggested above, this process involves each of the students telling the story of their painting to the whole group. In view of this, it is important to recognise how the group functions. How the individual and group connect with each other will have a bearing on offering each other the opportunity for stepping into the story. A group that is made up of individuals who have the ability to be there for others and are able to give recognition of shared similar experiences and emotions will gain enormously from this approach to education. However, it is paramount that the teacher(s) recognises the vulnerabilities of the individual students and of the group they belong to.

In promoting inclusion across the group, once all the students have completed their paintings we ask each of the students in turn to tell their story to the group. The depth of information the student is willing to divulge and/or their ability to talk in front of the group will impact on the time taken by each student. Our experience has been that allowing 5–8 minutes for each story will give some indication of the time needed for the session. Talking to a peer group of anything from 10 to 25 students can be a daunting task for the student hence we would reiterate sensitivity and caring on the part of the educationalist. In addition, and as previously stated, we would also suggest that two teachers work with a group of no more than 25 students. Whilst questions will need to be asked with regard to the painting, these must be framed in a supportive way that also encourages the student when answering to explore their own painting. It is important that the teacher uses his/her skill at being able to judge how far to take the individual and the group through alternative readings of the painting and which connecting theories would be most applicable and helpful to the student in the light of what they are presenting.

For both the student nurses and the authors (as educationalists), exploring these felt experiences proved to be rich in opportunity for reflection, reflexivity and contextualising self in relation to others. These were important opportunities for the student nurses to recognise the impact of self-awareness and reflexive practice on the quality of patient experience.

■ Conclusion

Education that ignores the value and development of emotions is one that denies the very heart of health and social care practice (Freshwater and Stickley, 2004). If teachers pay little attention to the emotional development of the student then they are likely to communicate to the student a lack of significance with regard to the interpersonal relationships they encounter in their everyday practice. In providing education that stimulates enquiry into one's emotional world, knowledge that is unknown and/or at times unspeakable can be brought safely into conscious awareness.

Personalising the educational process through art as a creative experiential learning focuses on the learning experience, thus requiring the student to explicate a level of enquiry and self-evaluation that will enable them to reach new understandings in terms of self and of their practice. When asked to paint their clinical experiences the visual drawing of such stimulates and challenges the student's thought process. In describing and therefore disclosing a number of factors through symbolic representation, these can then be progressed on to verbal expressions of meaning and understanding. As symbolic representation arises as more immediate raw knowledge, it has the potential to lead to making sense of thoughts and feelings that the student associates with that particular encounter (Lett, 1995). Through the verification of these understandings via interactive dialogue between the teacher, the student and the rest of their peer group translating the expressed experience into learning possibilities, the emotional context of their experience will be enhanced. Furthermore, through the validation of such personal and professional experience the important component of emotionality will become integral to the educational process.

References

Bateman, A. and Holmes, J. (1995) *Introduction to Psychoanalysis.* Routledge: London.

Berne, E. (1961) *Transactional Analysis in Psychotherapy.* Grove Press: New York.

Freshwater, D. and Stickley, T. (2004) The heart of art: Emotional intelligence in nurse education. *Nursing Inquiry,* 11 (2), 91–98.

Gilmartin, J. (2000) Psychodynamic sources of resistance among student nurses: Some observations in a human relations context. *Journal of Advanced Nursing,* 32 (6), 1533–1541.

Goldberg, C. (1993) The unexplored in self analysis. *Psychotherapy,* 30 (1), 159–161.

Hochschild, A.R. (1983) *The Managed Heart.* University of California Press: California.

Lett, W. (1995) Experiential supervision through simultaneous drawing and talking. *The Arts in Psychotherapy,* 22 (4), 315–328.

Mann, D. (2006) Art Therapy: Re-imagining a psychoanalytic perspective – A reply to David Maclagan. *International Journal of Art Therapy,* 11 (1), 33–40.

Nolan, M., Owen, G. and Nolan, J. (1995) Continuing professional education: Identifying characteristics of an effective system. *Journal of Advanced Nursing,* 22, 221–556.

Rogers, N. (1993) *The Creative Connection.* Science and Behaviour Books: California.

Scott, G. (2003) Has nursing lost its heart? *Nursing Standard,* 18 (13), 12–13.

Searle, J.T. (1992) Researching the other/searching for self: Qualitative research on [homo]sexuality in education. *Theory into Practice,* 31 (2, Spring), 147–156.

Warne, T. and McAndrew, S. (2005a) Political correctness, therapeutic naivety: The furtive future of primary mental health care. *Journal of Primary Mental Health Care,* 3 (1), 19–25.

Warne, T. and McAndrew, S. (2005b) The shackles of abuse: Unprepared to work at the edges of reason? *Journal of Psychiatric and Mental Health Nursing,* 12, 679–685.

Warne, T. and McAndrew, S. (2006) Splitting the difference: The heroes and villains of mental health policy and nursing practice. *Issues in Mental Health Nursing,* 27 (9), 1001–1013.

Chapter 10

Cinematic health and social care: Developing empathy and connecting with the screen experience

Gary Morris

■ Introduction

This chapter explores the value of using feature films within classroom teaching for facilitating the development of empathy. Film is a dynamic resource that helps to develop understanding as well as shape attitudes and feelings about those experiencing a myriad of health and social care problems (King and Watson, 2005; Mason, 2003; Morris, 2006). It should be noted here that this is intended as a complementary approach, to be used in tandem with other learning strategies which help develop empathy. There are many cinematic examples which can be used by educationalists to help students and practitioners appreciate the experience of illness. For example, *I am Sam* and *Rain Man* focused on learning disability; cancer is addressed in *Champions* and *Ikiru*; disfigurement in *The Elephant Man* and *Mask*; cerebral palsy in *My Left Foot*; physical disability in *Born on the 4th July* and *The Sea Inside*; AIDS in *Touch Me*; epilepsy in *First Do No Harm*; transplantation in *21 Grams*; drug abuse in *Trainspotting* and *Blow*; ADHD in *Thumbsucker*; child health/development in *Secret of the Wild Child* and *About a Boy*; older-adult care in *The Notebook*; terminal illness in *Terms of Endearment* and *Love Story*; and domestic violence/abuse in *The Prince of Tides* and *The Color Purple*. As these examples illustrate, the cinematic world provides viewers with a wealth of material concerning health and illness. If selected carefully these can act as a valuable guide as to the impact that various conditions and illnesses have upon individuals' lives and the types of care received from professionals and informal carers. Significant learning follows when the students are given the opportunity to discuss and process their findings with others.

Film is a very attractive and engaging medium which has significant learning potential. Indeed, I have noted the sense of excitement and enthusiasm demonstrated by learners when it is announced that 'we are about to watch a film'. It is a medium which has lasting appeal as images and characters served up to audiences can continue to resonate many years after their initial exposure (Welch and Racine, 1999). Film has the capacity to influence our understanding and awareness through the diverse selection of characters and events we are exposed to. Whilst this includes some very potent and memorable examples of people's struggles with health problems or disability (*The Elephant Man*; *A Beautiful Mind*), the environment of care (*Iris*; *Girl Interrupted*) and the cathartic breakthrough (*Good Will Hunting*; *Philadelphia*), it can also portray illness as a comedic (*Carry on Nurse*; *The Dream Team*) or frightening (*A Silence of the Lambs*; *Trainspotting*) entity. The accuracy and sensitivity of the material being portrayed will obviously vary with both good and poor examples being found. It is not necessarily the case that educationalists will simply opt for the more positive products as even misleading or stereotypical content can promote effective learning if challenged and discussed within an educational milieu.

A number of films have been used by me in teaching sessions with nursing and medical students and include *Some Voices*, *Iris* and *Awakenings*. These films have been found to be an engaging and stimulating means of 'tuning' students in to the service-user's world. It is not always essential to show films in their entirety as this can be very time-intensive and specifically selected clips – for example, Bob Champion's receipt of his cancer diagnosis in the film *Champions* – might serve to illustrate a point and promote discussion. It is the showing of the whole film *Some Voices*, though, which is to be used as an example in this chapter. This film has been used by me on a number of occasions and has evoked significant discussion amongst learners. The film portrays schizophrenia and offers an opportunity to appreciate something of the actual lived and felt experience of those afflicted with this condition.

■ Teaching empathy and connecting skills

One of the most fundamental skills required within health and social care practice is the ability to connect with the 'felt' world of those we are caring for. It is a process which has been written about extensively through such terms as 'empathy', 'identification' and 'engagement', but there appears to be no conclusive evidence that existing courses help health and social care professionals learn to show empathy. To address this, a concerted effort is required in both clinical and classroom settings (Reynolds, 2000).

The process of empathy was described clearly and succinctly by Carl Rogers (1951:29) as

> The ability of the therapist to sense the client's private world as if it were their own.

This definition strongly reflects the process of identification, whereby one is able to achieve a sense of shared perspective or, in essence, connect with and appreciate how things appear from another person's unique vantage point as if we ourselves were in their position. A particular problem with this definition is the phrasing

> ... as if it were their own.

As each person has their own personal set of experiences and unique way of looking at the world, it means that we may struggle when trying to apply our particular frame of reference to that of others. For example, a person's severe grief reaction over the loss of a favoured pet may seem to us to be extreme and out of context with the actual experience. We may have had a *similar* experience when we felt sad and which took a while to come to terms with although we were enabled, perhaps with the help of a replacement pet, to move on. What we can potentially miss here is the significance of what we might consider to be a 'minor bereavement' means or represents to another person. It might, for example, mean the loss of that individual's sole companion or trigger feelings of intense sadness associated with past unresolved losses. What we are looking at therefore is an ability to approach others with a much more receptive and open-minded approach regarding what their experiences might represent or signify in their totality.

One of the challenges facing educators is that of facilitating the learning and development of empathic approaches. Reynolds (2000) aired concerns whereby professional helpers are found to be only displaying low levels of empathy. If this is to be addressed, attention to educational activities is needed, as it appears that the theoretical grasp of such concepts is not being borne out by actual practice ability. Therefore, whilst students write at length within academic assignments about the feelings and personal experience of those experiencing health problems, evidence suggests that they find it difficult to actually connect with these aspects on an emotional as well as a cognitive level. Certain barriers to such integration are well documented in the literature (Reynolds, 2002; Warne and McAndrew, 2005), not least the feelings of discomfort experienced through close proximity to another person's distress.

Perhaps the prime location for developing empathy is the clinical setting with its opportunities for patient contact, clinical supervision and personal reflection. Whilst this is arguably the most potent means of developing insightful understanding, it has its limitations as we engage with the person out of the context provided by their usual day-to-day life. For example, within the protective space provided by a clinical setting the individual may appear relaxed and safe in the knowledge that their health needs are being addressed, yet in their home environment signs of illness-related stress may become exacerbated. Hearing about this stress from the person's recollections is very different to actually observing them in the midst of encountering these feelings. Other significant teaching approaches for developing empathy are outlined in other chapters. They include experiential learning and simulated patient work (Chapter 5); literature and poetry (Chapter 8); painting (Chapter 9); and, as put forward in this chapter, the medium of film. Non-clinical approaches help to build upon the totality of what is learnt or not learnt in practice. Such innovative approaches can offer valuable learning opportunities by enabling educationists to help guide learning as well as provide students with a safe space to discuss thoughts and feelings with peers.

■ Film and teaching

The medium of film provides learners with a rich communication source combining dialogue and music with visual imagery. It is a medium which is becoming much more prominent within the field of education; for example, psychology (Fleming et al., 1990) and the teaching of languages (Koch and Dollarhide, 2000). Over the past decade, its use within health care teaching has been increasing with its recognition as an effective and important learning resource for medicine (Zerby, 2005; Bhugra, 2003a) and nursing (Bag, 2004; Raingruber, 2003).

The importance of film as an aid to education is outlined by Ber (2001) through the utilisation of what are termed 'trigger' films. The 'trigger' film is a specifically produced short film whose aim is to stimulate and provoke learning (Nichols, 1994). Whilst these films might be created with an educational purpose in mind, well-chosen feature films may have similar impact on the student (Alexander, 2005; Raingruber, 2003).

An important attraction concerning the use of popular films is that unlike commercially produced educational material, they are relatively easy to access and can be more affordable. Also, students are likely to view these activities as exciting and innovative, thereby encouraging their participation (Diez et al., 2005). The engaging potential of film and its power to stimulate thought and discussion about health issues is reflected by various initiatives that have been piloted over the past few years. For example, film festivals have been set up covering themes as diverse as disability (Film London, 2005), transplantation (Wellcome Trust, 2006), women's health (UCSC, 2007), learning disability (Sprout, 2007), AIDS (New York AIDS Film Festival, 2007) and mental illness (*Reel Madness, Mind Odyssey* and

One in Four). The success of these events highlights the educational potential inherent in the medium of film. If allied with appropriate discussion, it is a core awareness-raising medium and one that is certainly well suited for the classroom.

There are a number of educational benefits that can be gained by health care professionals through making film recommendations to students as a means of developing understanding about specific health and social care topics (Hyler and Morre, 1996; Bhugra, 2003b). The selection and utilisation of films needs to be done with thought as to their appropriateness to what is being taught and the range of messages that might be accessed, particularly in the light of the distorting and stigmatising portrayal found within a large number of films. It is an approach, though, which furthers understanding of specific conditions, particularly where deficiencies in practice are noted. Alexander et al. (2005) found 'cinemeducation' important in teaching learners about depression and anxiety, two very common conditions that are related to numerous illnesses and affect large numbers of people. They cite the use of films such as *Ordinary People* and *Analyze This* as helpful resources for aiding learning.

One of the benefits from using film to help understand a person's inner world is the process of engaging in the present. This reflects the therapeutic process illustrated by Yalom (1995) of 'here and now' as opposed to 'there and then' as the observation and engagement of an individual's experience takes place immediately in front of the viewer. This takes the learning beyond isolated clinical encounters and provides learners with the understanding of how an individual experiences their symptoms in the context of their everyday lives (Bhugra, 2003a), thus experiencing the magical world of film as a better way to understand the requirements of the caring process (Frisch, 2001).

■ Empathising with the screen character

Films can be immensely engaging and can evoke a diverse range of feelings from their viewers. Although we know that most screen characters are, in essence, fictional constructs (apart from the biopic or documentary film), we still find ourselves responding with various emotions to the events occurring before us. Different types of film will evoke different feelings for different people. For example, I experienced fear and unsettlement when observing Norman Bates' murderous antics (*Psycho*), whilst I felt sympathy and sadness towards Iris Murdoch when seeing her distressing deterioration (*Iris*). It is this latter type which is most instrumental in developing empathy – where our emotions are engaged with what others might be experiencing or feeling. It is not always an easy or necessarily comfortable experience as unfamiliar and unsettling feelings might emerge.

This can reflect the strangeness or uniqueness of what we are experiencing as the related thoughts and feelings or level of distorted cognition found with some types of illnesses are hard for us to contemplate. It is the expressive and creative skill of the director allied with our imaginative ability that combines to foster new awareness and understanding. It relies, though, in part upon a 'suspension of belief' occurring whereby viewers imagine themselves to be the character with whom they are identifying with (Gaut, 2006). Of course this has its limitations as particular factors place a screen character's experience in a context that is alien to us by virtue of factors such as historical era, gender issues, cultural considerations or type of illness. Therefore we do not *know* what another person's experience feels like and can only *imagine.* Currie (1995) argues that if identification occurred in the *point of view shot* (showing what a character is looking at) then viewers would have to imagine that what happens to the screen character also happens to them and that they have some concern or sympathy for that person. Some films are very skilful at handling this, such as Ron Howard's *A Beautiful Mind.* In this film the viewer is given their own experience of hallucinatory imagery and a sense of uncertainty between reality and fantasy as characters that are seen and heard, we later learn, are actually constructs of Nash's disordered thoughts. In one striking scene, the perspective switches rapidly between John Nash's viewpoint and that of the crowd surrounding him. The emotions we feel are influenced by whichever perspective is offered as we alternatively see his anguish and agitation as he is taunted and harangued by Parcher, the government agent (Nash's viewpoint) or simply a 'madman' flailing about and shouting at the voices only he hears (the crowd's viewpoint).

■ The medium of film

A film narrative is constructed from a series of interrelated events, characters and actions out of which the audience creates a larger fictional world (Neupert, 1999). It is a very accessible and appealing medium which has the potential to engage audience members in more than simply a passive reception role. Here the viewer becomes an active participant in the process, being encouraged to enter into what Wedding and Boyd (1999) regard as a type of dissociative state where ordinary everyday existence is temporarily suspended. We have a sense of the camera superseding our own viewing perspective as we collapse the distinction between our eyes and the projection apparatus (Metz, 1982). Therefore, for the ninety or so minutes of a film's duration we are drawn into the enticing world set out before us and stimulated towards forming a real emotional attachment to the characters and situations being portrayed, having a sense of 'belief' in what we are observing.

Within the process the viewer is an active participant, engaging with the illusion offered yet at the same time able to retain a measure of detachment (Carroll, 1988). Whilst this to a degree might apply, there will be a number of occasions where viewers struggle to distinguish between reality and fiction. This is especially concerning given the proliferation of stereotypes and misrepresentations such as the idea that mentally ill people pose a serious threat to the general public or the belief that schizophrenia is synonymous with the condition of split personality. This is where opportunities for subsequent discussion and reflection help develop proper awareness and understanding.

It is also worth bearing in mind that each viewer will have their own separate interpretation of what they are watching, and the surface *verisimilitude* will differ from one member of the audience to another (Armstrong, 2005). From a mental health perspective we can consider the discrepancies between what is observed and understood by health care professionals and patients and those of general members of the public. This is borne out by largely successful and popular films such as *Me, Myself and Irene* which have been poorly reviewed by mental health advocates such as Mind, the National Schizophrenia Fellowship and the Royal College of Psychiatrists (Mind, 2000). In this film Jim Carrey shifts between two separate personality states: mentally well, mild-mannered Charlie; and mentally ill, offensive Hank. If watched in a learning situation, there are opportunities to challenge the inaccurate content as well as to consider what the impact might be upon resultant understanding and attitudes. For some learners it might involve re-looking at a product that was accessed at an earlier point but now scrutinised for new understanding. For example, we might have previously been greatly entertained and amused by Jim Carrey's antics and manic gesturing yet now hold an awareness of the potential damage caused through the perpetuation of age-old stereotypes.

Therefore, film can be regarded as having great learning potential. The need, though, is to be aware of what interpretations are being made and the resultant thoughts and feelings taken away. We will now look specifically at the use of the film *Some Voices*, including the preparation of learners and resultant discussion and debriefing.

☐ *Some Voices*

The film *Some Voices* follows Ray's (Daniel Craig) attempts at coping in the community following his discharge from hospital. The main focus is upon Ray's experience of schizophrenia and the relationship that he has with his brother Pete (Dave Morrissey) and his girlfriend Laura (Kelly Macdonald). It is a very powerful illustration of how different individuals perceive and cope with the experience of mental illness and the difficulties they face.

There are many films available depicting the condition and experience of schizophrenia covering the entire spectrum from the sensitive and informative through to the overly dramatic and extremely poor. *Some Voices* fits in with the better type of film as, unlike many other screen depictions about schizophrenia, the film fosters a feeling of caring. It portrays the condition accurately and avoids the traditionally confusing and misrepresented stereotypes. There is some violence perpetrated by Ray against another character, but in the context of his whole experience we the audience are able to understand what emotions and issues this behaviour is fuelled by. It is a film which provides a strong sense of Ray's mental health state from both a *felt* and *lived* perspective and facilitates an understanding of the 'experience' of schizophrenia and its consequent impact upon relationships.

Another factor in the selection of this film is the fact that the central character with mental health problems is also likeable and engaging. Although not boasting a top-bill cast at the time of its release, it nevertheless features some creditable and respected actors. It is interesting to watch the film now in terms of what we know about its primary star – Daniel Craig. On a showing of this film to a group of students a week after the general release of *Casino Royale* some surprised and pleased remarks were noted – 'Oh look it's James Bond.' This certainly helps with a core intention of showing the film to students – to feature a person with mental health problems who is likeable and attractive, very different from the stereotype reinforced through many other media products.

The 'typical' portrayal features largely unappealing individuals whom the audience struggle to warm to. The concept of *liking* is important as it plays a significant role in the type of emotional response evoked in the audience; for example, feeling concern for a person's welfare (Hoffner and Cantor, 1991). Recent years have heralded a greater use of charismatic and appealing stars with the *experience* of illness starting to take precedence over a person's actions. Examples of positive role models include Judy Dench (*Iris*), Meryl Streep (*Sylvia*) and Tom Hanks (*Philadelphia*). A particularly important association concerns the collective positive attributes that such likeable and charismatic stars carry with them; for example, the view that physically attractive people are regarded as possessing more socially desirable personality traits than those deemed unattractive (Hatfield and Sprecher, 1986). There is also the view that liked characters encourage viewers to identify with and vicariously experience what they are going through (Zillman, 1980). What is significant here is the distancing from traditionally held views and the opportunity to question and challenge one's own feelings about those with more stigmatised health problems. The selection, therefore, of *Some Voices* and Daniel Craig's performance offers viewers an appealing person with mental health issues, someone who appears and looks *normal* and who is largely engaged in *ordinary* activities.

☐ *Critical receipt*

This film on the whole has been critically well received and stands out from the plethora of mental health–related films as one of the more sensitive and thoughtful portrayals (see Box 10.1).

Box 10.1: What the critics said

'A sympathetic and substantial depiction of schizophrenia' (Peter Bradshaw – Guardian Unlimited 2000).

'Some Voices is a welcome, thoughtful, and engaging film – at last, a film that rises above the usual dross of mental illness movies' (Peter Byrne – British Medical Journal 2000).

'...the heart of the film, the relationship between the brothers, is wonderfully full, and Ray's instability is capably reflected in the uncertainty and random violence of Shepherd's Bush' (Michael Thompson – BBC 2000).

'Outstanding cerebral London-based drama about a schizophrenic dealing with life in the community – and the community dealing with him – on his discharge from psychiatric hospital' (Channel 4 2000).

'Unambitious small scale drama concentrating on a fractured relationship between the two brothers. Despite the creditable performances it would seem best suited for the TV movie "disease of the week"' (Halliwell's Film Guide 2007).

'Definitely worth seeing, showcases some terrific British talent and only fails to make the four star grade by a whisker' (Mark Wyman's Film Review – also in Halliwell's Film Guide 2007).–

☐ *Watching the film*

The approach taken is of asking students to reflect upon key questions at designated points before, during and after viewing the film (see Box 10.2). This enables them to consider the impact that the screen portrayal has upon them.

Box 10.2: Film worksheet

Before:
- *What is schizophrenia?*
- *What do you feel might be a person's felt or lived experience of schizophrenia?*
- *Where does your current understanding come from?*

During:
Please jot down any thoughts or aspects relating to the questions
below as you watch the film.

- *In what ways do you see Ray being affected by his mental health state?*
- *How does his brother Pete cope with it?*
- *What is the impact upon Ray's relationships with his girlfriend Laura?*
- *What are your feelings with regards to Ray?*

After:

- *What do we learn about the experience of Schizophrenia from this film?*

1) Before:

- What is schizophrenia?
- What do you feel might be a person's felt or lived experience of
  schizophrenia?
- Where does your current understanding come from?

The first questions relate to current understanding and apply equally to
students at any level of knowledge or experience. The importance here is
of establishing a focal point from which to reflect upon whilst watching the
film. Students are asked to consider what they know about schizophrenia
as well as where they have learnt their information from. This might be
from clinical practice, classroom teaching, reading, personal experience or
media products they have been exposed to. It is worth noting, though, that
we continuously experience competing stimuli and may find it hard to separate out all of the associated learning. For example, the more empathic
and informed learning from clinical practice might be offset by media
products that 'tell' us that the 'mentally ill' are highly likely to be violent
towards themselves or others. Teasing out common misperceptions (i.e.
psychotic = psychopathic or the overestimated violence potential) is part of
the process and it is important to stress to students to feel free at this stage
to write without concern over what the 'right' answers might be. The initial questions therefore set a base for students and help to tune them in to
the theme being addressed. It is something to look at later to help evaluate
and review learning and reflects the processes illustrated by Kolb's experiential learning cycle (Kolb, 1984) or Gibbs' model of reflection (Gibbs,
1988). These show learning being generated through a series of events
whereby reflection and experience follow each other in succession, each
influenced in turn by the quality of the preceding dynamics. Having written
answers to these questions, it is useful to provide opportunities for students
to share their initial thoughts with others before proceeding to watching
the film.

2) During:

- In what ways do you see Ray being affected by his mental health state?
- How does his brother Pete cope with it?
- What is the impact upon Ray's relationship with his girlfriend Laura?
- What are your feelings with regard to Ray?

There are some very potent illustrations within this film that help viewers appreciate something of Ray's personal experience, including his thoughts and feelings. One scene in particular reflects his feelings of paranoia whilst walking through a London marketplace. The dissociated images and sounds, coupled with a selection of fleeting impressions (being stared at, a remark chalked on the pavement, a plastic gun on a market stall) all work at giving the viewer a sense of Ray's tension and unease. Instead of look- ing at this experience from a purely objective distance (i.e. simply seeing a person behaving oddly), we the viewers are provided with an emotional connection and a sense of what it feels like. Watching this film gives us a number of such examples and traces Ray's progress through a series of highs and lows. Viewers are shown glimpses of his corresponding emotions such as confusion, elation, fear, contentment, agitation and sadness. Chart- ing this progress means that we are better able to understand the 'total' experience and understand how an individual experiences their symptoms in the context of their daily lives and not solely through isolated clinical encounters.

Pete (his brother) clearly struggles to cope with Ray's increasingly erratic behaviour and reflects something of the conflict and stress endured by many carers or family members of those experiencing schizophrenia (Rethink, 2007). The conflict is reflected in Pete's response to Ray, who on the whole is supportive and caring although becomes rejecting and frus- trated as various pressures takes their toll. Pete provides a sharp contrast to Ray's girlfriend Laura. Whilst Pete is conventional and quickly irritated by Ray's erratic behaviour, Laura is more free-spirited and able to cele- brate and be engaged by his quirkiness. All this gives the viewer a sense of how some people struggle when met with approaches which are per- sonally restrictive or stifling. Laura provides Ray with a sense of freedom, reminiscent of the expressive creativity found in a number of celebrated artists (i.e. Salvador Dali). Here quirky or eccentric expression has an out- let, a value and sense of acceptance rather than being met with restriction or dismissal. The sense we gain therefore is something of how the responses from others can either exacerbate a person's problems making them feel unduly stressed and restricted or alternatively providing feelings of free- dom and greater acceptance. What we do see clearly is the stress that mental health problems can place upon relationships. It is a process high- lighted by Barham and Hayward (1991) as strongly influencing a sense of disconnection or feelings of social isolation.

Our feelings towards Ray are influenced by gaining a greater awareness of what he is experiencing internally. This is aided through the style of production as well as some very believable and strong central performances. Whilst watching some of the scenes, the *mise-en-scène* (camerawork) shows us the world as seen through Ray's eyes and we are manipulated towards his inner world whereby we feel some of his suspicion and paranoia. Our engagement is facilitated through this 'knowledge' of what is occurring internally as well as being presented with a largely attractive and likeable character. This contrasts with the often-depicted strange or creepy-looking person that forms Wahl's concept of the mentally ill as a 'breed apart' (Wahl, 1995). Portrayals such as this are important because of helping viewers firstly to identify with screen characters and secondly to develop a sense of actually caring about them.

3) After:

• What do we learn about the experience of Schizophrenia from this film?

This stage is the processing section whereby students' initial views can be revisited and new learning encouraged. It has been notable that whilst most students subsequently tend to view the condition of schizophrenia more favourably, others find it hard to ignore the film's more violent scenes. The different interpretation can partly be explained through perceptual theories such as Gestalt theory whereby elements that stand out (*figure and ground*) are strongly influenced by a person's previous knowledge and experience (Köhler, 1930).

Empathising with fictional characters involves *imagining* what their beliefs and desires might be. We are given some indication of this although we are still unable to check things out. What we have in a sense is still an experience largely governed by what we imagine we might feel if in another's position. What is perhaps important with the example from *Some Voices* is not necessarily having to understand exactly what Ray might be feeling and experiencing but having a more thoughtful and questioning outlook and being able to transfer this understanding to others with this condition within our sphere of care. This certainly seems to fit with the general thoughts and feelings of students subsequent to viewing this film.

■ Conclusion

The cinematic world has much learning potential to offer health care students. The example related here concerns that of schizophrenia although the process can equally be applied to many other themes where film examples are available. We need not necessarily search for 'perfect' examples as both positive and negative components are able to generate thoughtful discussion. The essence of this process is the degree of guidance and discussion afforded to students to help make sense of interpretations. Educationalists interested in using films should therefore be mindful of the whole process; for example, the relevance of what is being shown, preparation of students for this process and opportunities to examine new learning taking place. A template for showing films within health and social care education is provided in Box 10.3. Whilst the primary example given here concerns a mental health issue there is no reason why the same process cannot be applied to any other health and social care theme. What is important is finding films that relate appropriately to health and social care issues that students are currently learning about or encountering in practice. The Appendix at the end of the book may help with this. Learning can be stimulated on multiple levels, including the focus upon a featured condition, various approaches to care or the impact that all of this has upon individuals' lives. With sufficient preparation, careful selection and supportive processing the cinematic world can be regarded as an immensely valuable and vibrant resource for learning.

Box 10.3: Showing films

Selecting films

Considerations:
- chosen film appropriately relates to an identified learning theme
- film is accessible
- appropriate educational licence is possessed to actually show the film
- am I showing the whole film or selected clips?
- appreciation as to what is good or bad about this film
- appropriateness of age rating to student group

Understanding of the film being shown

Awareness of the messages being conveyed:
- characterisation
- relationships
- imagery
- dialogue
- sound and music
- environment/background features

Student preparation

- introduction of students to learning topic
- drawing up of related questions/worksheet
- (if necessary), give students warning of content; that is, swearing, nudity or violence

---

Processing

- opportunities for feedback and discussion
- follow-up and consolidation
- direct students towards other resources (i.e. other films, books or Internet sites)

References

Alexander, M. (2005). A graduate survey of cinemeducation. In Alexander, M., Lenahan, P. and Pavlov, A. (eds.) *Cinemeducation. A Comprehensive Guide to using Film in Medical Education.* Abingdon: Radcliffe Publishing, pp. 184–187.

Alexander, M., Waxman, D. and Simpson, J. (2005). Anxiety, depression and somatoform disorders. In Alexander, M., Lenahan, P. and Pavlov, A. (eds.) *Cinemeducation. A Comprehensive Guide to Using Film in Medical Education.* Abingdon: Radcliffe Publishing, pp. 82–87.

Armstrong, R. (2005). *Understanding Realism.* London: British Film Institute.

Bag, B. (2004). Einsatz von Spielfilmen in der Ausbildung von Krankenpfegern in der Psychiatrie am Beispiel des Spielfilms "Iris". *PrinterNet.* 10, 521–525.

Barham, P. and Hayward, R. (1991). *From the Mental Patient to the Person.* London: Routledge.

Ber, R. (2001). Twenty years of experience using trigger films as a teaching tool. *Academia Medica.* 76, 656–658.

Bhugra, D. (2003a). Teaching psychiatry through cinema. *Psychiatric Bulletin.* 27, 429–430.

Bhugra, D. (2003b). Using film and literature for cultural competence training. *Psychiatric Bulletin.* 27, 427–428.

Carroll, N. (1988). *Mystifying Movies. Fads and Fallacies in Contemporary Film Theory.* New York: Columbia University Press.

Currie, G. (1995). *Image and Mind: Film Philosophy and Cognitive Science.* Cambridge: Cambridge University Press.

Diez, K., Pleban, F. and Wood, R. (2005). Teaching techniques. Lights, camera, action: Integrating popular film in the health classroom. *Journal of School Health.* 75(7), 271–275.

Film London (2005). Disability Film Festival. Available at http://www.filmlondon. org.uk/news_details.asp?NewsID=261 (Accessed 17 December 2007).

Fleming, M., Piedmont, R. and Hiam, C. M. (1990). Images of madness: feature films in teaching psychology. *Teaching of Psychology,* 17, 185–187.

Frisch, L. (2001). Friday night at the movies. In Frisch, N. and Frisch, L. (eds.) *Psychiatric Mental Health Nursing.* Albany, NY: Delmar Publishers. pp. 779–799.

Gaut, B. (2006). Identification and emotion in narrative film. In Carroll, N. and Choi, J. (eds.) *Philosophy of Film and Motion Pictures.* Oxford: Blackwell Publishing. pp. 260–270.

Gibbs, G. (1988). *Learning by Doing: A Guide to Teaching and Learning Methods.* London: FEU.

Hatfield, E. and Sprecher, S. (1986). *Mirror, Mirror... The Importance of Looks in Everyday Life.* New York: State University of New York Press.

Hoffner, C. and Cantor, J. (1991). Perceiving and responding to mass media characters. In Bryant, J. and Zillman, D. (eds.) *Responding to the Screen: Reception and Reaction Process.* New Jersey: Lawrence Erlbaum Associates. pp. 63–101.

Hyler, S. and Morre, J. (1996). Teaching psychiatry? Let Hollywood help! Suicide in the cinema. *Academic Psychiatry.* 20(4), 212–219.

King, M. and Watson, K. (2005). *Representing Health: Discourses of Health and Illness in the Media.* Basingstoke: Palgrave Macmillan.

Koch, G. and Dollarhide, C. (2000). Using a popular film in counsellor education. *Counselor Education and Supervision.* 39, 203–211.

Köhler, W. (1930). *Gestalt Psychology.* London: G. Bell.

Kolb, D. (1984). *Experiential Learning: Experience as the Source of Learning and Development.* London: Prentice Hall.

Mason, G. (2003). News media portrayal of mental illness: Implications for public policy. *American Behavioural Scientist.* 46(12), 1594–1600.

Metz, C. (1982). *The Imaginary Signifier: Psychoanalysis and the Cinema.* Bloomington: Indiana University Press.

Mind (2000). *Me, Myself and Irene.* Available at http://www.mind.org.uk/News+ policy+and+campaigns/Press+archive/Mental+Health+Groups+Unite+to+ Criticise+New+Carrey+Comedy.htm (Accessed 22nd March 2007).

Morris, G. (2006). *Mental Health Issues and the Media.* London: Routledge.

Neupert, R. (1999). Theoretical frameworks: Looking at film. In Cook, P. and Bernink, M. (eds.) *The Cinema Book.* (2nd ed). London: British Film Institute, pp. 319–323.

Nichols, J. (1994). The trigger film in nurse education. *Nurse Education Today.* 14(4), 326–330.

Raingruber, B. (2003). Integrating aesthetics into advanced practice mental health nursing: Commercial film as a suggested modality. *Issues in Mental Health Nursing.* 24(5), 467–495.

Rethink (2007). *Living with Mental Illness.* Available at http://www.rethink.org/ living_with_mental_illness/index.html/ (Accessed 23rd November 2007).

Reynolds, W. (2000). *The Measurement and Development of Empathy in Nursing.* Aldershot: Ashgate.

Reynolds, P. (2002). The role of avoidance. *British Medical Journal.* 324, 857.

Rogers, C. (1951). *Client-Centered Therapy: Its Current Practice, Implications and Theory.* London: Constable.

Sprout (2007). Sprout Film Festival. Available at http://www.gosprout.org/film/ (Accessed 16 December 2007).

UCSC (2007). Lunafest Film Festival. Available at http://currents.ucsc.edu/06- 07/01-22/brief-lunafest.asp (Accessed 10 December 2007).

Wahl, O. (1995). *Media Madness: Public Images of Mental Illness.* New Jersey: Rutgers University Press.

Warne, T. and McAndrew, S. (2005). The shackles of abuse: Unprepared to work at the edges of reason. *Journal of Psychiatric and Mental Health Nursing,* 12, 679–686.

Wedding, D. and Boyd, M. (1999). *Movies and Mental Illness.* Boston, MA: McGraw Hill Education.

Welch, M. and Racine, T. (1999). A psycho for every generation. *Nursing Inquiry.* 6(3), 216–219.

Wellcome Trust (2006). The ethics of transplantation. Available at http://www. wellcome.ac.uk/doc_WTX034323.html (Accessed 12 December 2007).

Yalom, I. (1995). *The Theory and Practice of Group Psychotherapy.* (4th edn). New York: Basic Books.

Zerby, S. (2005). Using the science fiction film *Invaders from Mars* in a child psychiatry seminar. *Academic Psychiatry.* 29, 316–321.

Zillman, D. (1980). Anatomy of suspense. In Tannenbaum, P. (ed.) *The Entertainment Functions of Television.* Hillsdale, NJ: Lawrence Erlsbaum. pp. 133–163.

Chapter 11

Awake and aware: Thinking constructively about the world through Transformative Learning

Margaret McAllister

■ Introduction

It was the final session of a three-week learning module in which students learned textual analysis and analysed representations of mental illness in film and literature. In addition to seeking written evaluations, I asked students in the class to give me feedback on how they found the learning. John, a charismatic and bright young man, piped up moaning theatrically: 'I'll never be able to lie on the couch and just watch a movie ever again'.

Reading between the lines, and as suggested in the previous chapter, John was telling me that the process had awakened him to issues of inequity and unfairness and stimulated him to know that he had a lot of work to do in his professional career in reducing stigma towards mental illness.

John's comment exemplifies the aims of Transformative Learning – students are awakened to issues of injustice, aware of the effects of dominating forces on vulnerable or marginalised groups, and there is an experience of transformation, altering the perspective and habits of mind they use to understand and interact with the world in the future.

Transformative Learning in early childhood, middle, senior and higher education has been around for over 15 years. In a recent meta-review of educational research papers, Taylor (2007) stated that it is the most researched and discussed topic in the field of adult education. There is wide variation in approaches, but the common features in this learning are that it engages students in critical reflection, and discussion of relevant disorienting dilemmas that become a catalyst for change. Thus, it aims to develop constructive thinking skills, not just critical.

This chapter explores important components of Transformative Learning so that readers too become awake to and aware that dominant modes of teaching can be silencing and disempowering; teachers need to find ways to sensitise learners to issues that demand *all* of our attention; activities need to be *purposeful* so they activate learners to generate solutions to world problems and are relevant to practice.

■ Transformative learning: What it is and isn't

Whilst essential for safe individual client care, teaching students the *functions* and *techniques* of practice is unlikely to make much contribution to social change. Whilst is a necessary component in health and social education, technique-dominated learning is not sufficient for skilled professional practice in health and social care. Indeed, there are many who argue that technical knowledge is inherently conservative (Habermas, 1972; Gee and Lankshear, 1995) – it offers health assessment/treatment skills but is not good at engendering critical, imaginative and creative thinking. Social problems are likely to go unaddressed, thereby offering implicit support for the status quo.

An alternative is Transformative Learning, defined by O'Sullivan and Morrell (2002, p. 18) as one that involves

> experiencing a deep, structural shift in the basic premises of thought, feelings, and actions. It is a shift of consciousness that dramatically and irreversibly alters our way of being in the world. Such a shift involves our understanding of ourselves and our self-locations; our relationships with other humans and with the natural world; our understanding of relations of power in interlocking structures of class, race and gender; our body awarenesses, our visions of alternative approaches to living; and our sense of possibilities for social justice and peace and personal joy.

A social justice approach not only stems from but also generates *critical* perspectives on the macro-level relationships of power, labour and ideology. It involves individual and collaborative efforts to *change* curricula, raise questions about common practices and resist inappropriate decisions (Giroux, 2000). In relation to health professionals, the goals in this model of teaching are for learners to begin to recognise the social and cultural practices that support dominant systems of health and social care in society as well as reflect on and change *their* role in perpetuating forms of injustice.

■ Awake to the world

In his book *The collapse of globalism* John Ralston Saul (2005), philosopher and cultural critic, has argued provocatively that globalism has failed.

Globalism is the social and economic theory, emerging in the 1970s, that declares that free trade of goods, capital, ideas and people will lead to more wealth, freedom, peace and connection. However, the reality has been starkly different.

Despite the fact that worldwide communication pathways are vast, some countries have transformed and prospered, some borders between nations have dissolved with good effects, and there are many new and complicated cultural interconnections worldwide, there is a mounting backlash against globalisation. Ralston Saul sees it in the impoverishment of rural culture, the resurgence of nationalism and fundamentalism, the rise of militarism and the failure to eradicate poverty, violence, corruption and disease in the developing world. Even though resources are plentiful and there is no good reason why some groups should be flourishing and others in despair, there is actually *more* social disconnection, discrimination and violence, and economic exclusion.

Without preaching at students or frightening them with doom and gloom, it is possible to awaken them so that they see that they have a role in making a positive difference. Transformative Learning places equal emphasis on engaging the learner by cultivating relationships, and conveying and developing cognitive skills, so that learners are equipped with knowledge resources for the future. Mezirow (1991, 2000), the educationalist attributed with beginning the discourse of Transformative Learning, explained that as individuals are socialised into a group, such as a health profession, they acquire ways of looking at the world and these become taken for granted and unquestioned. Transformative Learning occurs when there is a transformation of a person's meaning structures, a perspective shift. Such a shift may be the result of a cumulative process, but often occurs as a consequence of a 'disorientating dilemma' that leads a person to critically reflect on the assumptions that underpin their meaning structures. It involves awareness that commonplace actions do not produce the expected results or fail to solve the problem.

To use nursing as an example, there are many disorientating dilemmas that are not effectively resolved using 'old' ways of thinking (Box 11.1).

Box 11.1: Disorientating dilemmas in nursing

- Nursing was once the care-based career, but now there are many. Nurses can no longer define themselves simply as the clinician who is there 24/7 and who provides nurture and comfort, for there are lifestyle attendants, social workers, disability support workers and so on.
- Workplace bullying is commented upon frequently, but it is also nothing new. Nursing has long been characterized as emerging from a top-down hierarchy where dominant leaders enforced

compliance with rules. Yet top-down leadership is disempowering and many nurses cite unwillingness to cope with being bossed and controlled as their reason for leaving.

- Duty and obedience once characterized the good nurse, and these virtues were and are valued over independent thinking and debate. Yet nursing preparation now occurs in a university setting where questioning and critical thinking are taught and valued. Educated women have other options open to them besides nursing and thus are not staying in nursing for their whole working career.
- The public once considered nursing an ideal trade for young girls with caring nature and a love of hard work. But cultural changes have opened up nursing to men and to advances in the science of human caring. Nurses learn that their work is complex and expanding, yet public perceptions minimise these changes and effectively constrain nursing's place in society.

■ When Transformative Learning is useful

Wherever social discrimination, injustice, disconnection, violence or other abuses of power occur, Transformative Learning has a place. Health topics that need a learner to be sensitised to the human impact of an issue and capable of generating new solutions include childhood neglect, domestic violence, indigenous health problems, youth, mental health, issues related to aging and social care, workplace bullying, migrants, refugees and other cross-cultural well-being issues, forensic health and survivors of trauma.

Readers can find examples of Transformative Learning approaches applied to topics as varied as environmental science, ethics, history, leadership, medical education, media studies, nursing, palliative care, peace and conflict studies, race relations and religion (Feinstein, 2004; Goldie et al., 2005; MacLeod et al., 2003). It has also been used with different types of learner groups such as those who are using English as a second language (King, 2000); learning online (Cragg et al., 2001); studying in an international country (Lyon, 2001), living with illness or disability (Baumgartner, 2002); or learning clinical education (McAllister, Tower and Walker, 2007).

■ Learning outcomes

The learning outcomes possible in this model of teaching and learning are many (Box 11.2). Foremost among them is that Transformative Learning changes perspective. This is crucial when learners don't care about a particular subject matter. Transformation in perspective may be needed to interrupt the tendency for such unhelpful attitudes to keep being reproduced and for the status quo to go unchallenged. Ideally, in the transformative classroom, students are enabled to clarify their life (professional and personal) mission and to live that life with purpose and direction.

Box 11.2: Learning outcomes

Changed perspective on self and others
- Anti-racist
- Pro-humanist
- Pro-justice
- Humble about difference
- Efficacious

Thinking skills
- More able questioners, challengers
- Critical, constructive thinkers
- More able to collectively solve problems

View of the future
- Hopeful
- Optimistic
- Visionary

Furthermore, because the transformative classroom makes a conscious effort to awaken and challenge students, cognitive outcomes include learners becoming more able questioners, critical and constructive thinkers, more self-directed, assertive and self-confident. Activities that are purposeful and relevant to the world of professional practice are also more likely to develop in students work-ready capabilities such as leadership, change and problem-solving. This also facilitates action, not just understanding around an issue.

Rather than the view to the future being fatalistic or pessimistic, because opportunities are created to discuss ideals and give students the faith that they can make a difference, learners are more likely to look ahead with optimism and self-efficacy.

Various educational research projects have produced evidence of positive effects on learners. In the context of media literacy, several studies have shown that it can produce measurable results in learners' ability to analyse, critique and produce media messages (Hobbs and Frost, 2003; Quin and McMahon, 1991). In the context of health professional learning, transformative approaches enhance empathy and understanding and prompt critical thinking, as well as the generation of alternative solutions to entrenched problems.

■ How to begin

It is important for teachers to *prepare* to teach transformatively, for this is an exercise in creative, energetic teaching that is unlike conventional styles. Just like the student, teachers need to consider how they have been socialised, to look again at commonplace practices that may have become naturalised and taken for granted – such as the tendency to fill the class time with delivery of content or assume the role of expert when students too may have expertise. Teachers, who are sensitive to the problems of domination and control, can set the tone for an inspiring, exciting, critical environment where new ideas and optimism for change prosper. I have written at length elsewhere on how to prepare for this novel teaching role (McAllister, 2005) and this involves attempts to engage students in a productive teaching relationship, and to build new cognitive and affective skills to help them build a better world. These strategies are summarised in Box 11.3 and Table 11.1. Key strategies will be elaborated on in turn.

Box 11.3: What do we NOT want the world to be?

- **A place where citizens do not see that they have the power to influence others.**
  So in the classroom, make it a place that is safe and trustworthy so that students learn that their opinions, experiences and perspectives when they are spoken and written have the power to influence others. *For example, set short activities that require each person's contribution and ensure that everyone's contribution is heard.*

- **A place where some people are so rich that they waste or hoard resources, pollute with their excesses, dominate and control, and others are so poor that they lack resources, are weak with hunger and disease, fight amongst themselves and are caught in a vicious self-harming cycle.**
  Discuss where this phenomenon occurs and make the class a place where students feel and are connected to those people fired up about power that excludes and economics matters more than people. *For example, invite consumers who have lived the experience to get to know the class and share their stories.*

- **A place where multinational corporations and big business wield power without comment, criticism or resistance.**
  Make the class a place where students learn that small business is a productive alternative. Changes at the local level make a difference.

For example, invite speakers who have implemented an innovation to share their success.

- **A place where individuals and groups feel alienated and despairing.** Create a place where students feel a sense of belonging, camaraderie and hope. *For example, ensure that constructive feedback is given and purposeful activities are set to show learners their potential to make a difference.*

- **A place where some people's misery is ignored, diminished, judged or set aside.** Cultivate responsibility for self and other is shared. This can be done by articulating group norms and making a decision about how to respond when the norms are transgressed. *For example, 'in this class when students feel left out, we will make an effort to involve them'.*

Table 11.1 Transformative teaching strategies

Nurturing the teacher–student relationship	Creating purposeful activities to	Building a critical consciousness, so that students
Acknowledge and appreciate difference.	Reveal inequities.	Release their imagination.
Form a partnership.	Disrupt the commonplace.	Clarify vision and values.
Explain the pedagogical approach.	Use many ways of knowing.	Self-interrogate habits, rituals and routines.
Voice the students.	Stimulate critical and constructive thinking.	Remember the value of knowing history.
Create space for dialogue – not just discussion.	Cultivate compassion.	Reveal and subvert the dominant paradigm.
Interrupt gently.		Claim practice linked with theory (rather than diminish its value).
		Listen to the voice of consumers.
		Are active in change projects.

☐   Release imagination

Although I never met her, Maxine Greene, the great educationalist and artist, is the teacher who most inspires me. In her classic book *Releasing the Imagination* Greene (1995, pp. 2–3) said that arousing imagination helps people to 'reach beyond [our present realities] … to some naming, some sense-making that brings us together in community'. She explained that wherever inequality and other dark experiences exist, art, music, poetry and other activities that draw on imagination can provide light, happiness and social connection (see Chapters 8 and 9 for using poetry and art). Imagination by its nature is about the uncertain. It invites people to reach beyond themselves and what is happening presently to what *might otherwise* be happening and what may be conceived as possible. This is the language of ideals.

In education programmes preparing students for professions there is a temptation to fill the curriculum with technical skills. Whilst practical classes have a valuable place they are also a site where the valorising of the 'real world' of practice diminishes a focus on the 'ideal world'. Emily Dickinson (1960, pp. 688–689) says this another way:

The possible's slow fuse is lit by the imagination!

Thus, whenever I'm preparing for classroom teaching or creating an online learning activity, I set myself the goal of arousing the learner's imagination – even if (or perhaps especially when) the topic seems straightforward, concrete or technical. For when the learner's imagination is awakened, they are engaged in the subject matter, and if this is paired with encouragement, patience and time, ideas begin to generate and flow and learners begin to see that they have the skills to critique and re-invent.

Frida Kahlo's paintings are a rich source for imagination exercises (cf. Herrera, 1991). Her painting of *The Little Deer* evokes much discussion on what it might be like to be marginalised, wounded, in pain and in need. It can also invite thinking on what the role of the engaged, committed, health professional could be in that encounter. When asked to imagine what the health professional could do in this image, students have offered suggestions such as to gently reorient the deer so that it turns towards the light and is thus able to see a way forward.

☐   Teach critical and constructive thinking

Assisting learners to release their imagination is one way to inspire constructive thinking – a skill that is slightly different from, and complementary to, critical thinking (Thayer-Bacon, 2000). Critical thinking is an ability to think deeply about an issue, and requires more than the ability to describe or recall. Where critical thinking very often involves deconstruction – a process of dismantling an issue so that its components are open to scrutiny and its devices revealed – constructive thinking involves reconstruction, a process where social problems are not just revealed, but solutions generated. Critical thinking has historically emphasised rational thinking – that which is dispassionate, deductive and science-based. Constructive thinking attempts to correct the imbalance in thinking about knowledge by arguing that human beings know things also through imagination, emotion and intuition and that deep thinking about an issue can be assisted through these artistic lenses.

Thus, in a transformative classroom, the objective is not to reject critical thinking, but to *augment* it, through constructive thinking exercises, such as those found in metaphor activities, poetry analysis and so on (see also Chapter 8), where the learner is assisted to imagine new ways of operating other than those that have been critiqued.

For example, after students have discussed the ethics in research I have used the metaphor of imagining the research field as a ruin. Students are shown an image of an archaeological dig and, once 'limbered up' cognitively, are asked to brainstorm ideas that are evoked about ways to conduct oneself ethically in research fields. Responses include that researchers need to carefully pick through data and details, taking care to suspend judgement and sustain a curious engagement with the field until it is time to draw conclusions; and it is important to notice how historical and present practices shape how practitioners operate (McAllister and Rowe, 2003). These are all constructive *and* critical ideas about research.

☐   Clarify vision and values

Students about to enter health and social care professions, or perhaps reflect on their place within it, can benefit from reflection on who 'we' are (as opposed to 'I'), what we stand for, and what we don't. As a member of a profession, identity is shared rather than simply personal, and thus there is value in spending time coming to know, feel and practise the shared values. Human development theories have shown that positive self-identity is strongly correlated with well-being, happiness, self-efficacy, internal locus of control and stress hardiness (Luthar, 2003). These are all characteristics of resilience. A focus on resilience rather than our weaknesses and troubles may assist in clarifying and strengthening professional identity. This is why as a teacher it is useful to spend time with students discussing what we stand for, what we believe in and what we might imagine doing differently.

Envisioning the world is sometimes easier when we reflect on what we don't want to see, or what we want to see no more of. It can also be a good way to establish class group norms and surface and clarify values.

☐   Interrupt gently

As has been explained, the process of socialisation within general society and the professional culture leads to the uptake and absorption of norms and ways of seeing the world that over time become deeply engrained and taken for granted. These tools of thinking are used often out of habit, rather than with conscious intent. When they are used inappropriately or ineffectively, the transformative teacher's role can be to interrupt them so that (a) they cannot occur without notice; and (b) an alternative way of thinking can be fostered.

A crucial mistake that I think humanistic teachers can sometimes make is when they nurture the student so much that no criticism is provided (Conway, 2001). In this case, learning is unlikely to occur, because the student is not taken out of their comfort zone and into the space where new learning takes place. So the transformative teacher has a role in identifying students at the edge of their knowing who need support to move into areas of unknowing, and this is frequently discomforting.

The easiest way to interrupt a student without them taking offence or losing face is to gain permission for this strategy in the forming stage of the teacher–student relationship. At the very first encounter with students, another important strategy of the transformative teacher can be employed – provide an explanation of the pedagogy that will shape the learning in this group. For example, the teacher could say, 'If I hear or see things that could be challenged, scrutinised or replaced, I will try to interrupt these with you. Is that OK?', and 'at what times will it not be ok?' This latter question, leads on to another point – that it is important to spend time giving voice to students.

☐   Find opportunities for students to interject their own voice

Parker Palmer (1998) once said that good teaching is 'an act of generosity' in that it takes a willingness to share, a lot of patience and persistence. Palmer writes so eloquently about the craft of teaching that readers are urged to find his books and articles and savour his wisdom directly (see the paper 'Good teaching: A matter of living the mystery' at http://teaching.uchicago.edu/pod/pod2/91-92/Palmer.htm).

Parker talks of patience and persistence because many students prefer to sit on the sidelines in silence. This, after all, is how many of us have been taught. Understandably, speaking up takes courage; there is a risk that others will criticise or even denigrate our ideas, yet when learners find their voice they also find power and influence. Ways to help students find their voice is to begin with issues that connect directly with their life and sparking learners' interest so that they *want* to speak. For example, rather than teach the mechanics of the heart via diagrams and talk, students could be taken on a quick run and asked to notice what changes were occurring in their body. Frequently I use excerpts from film, television, music or poetry and ask students to describe what they have just observed. Being able to describe is a relatively easy task. Gradually I make the task more challenging by teaching a cognitive skill, and asking the student to use that skill to interrogate the text.

Alternatively, when difficult topics arise, Palmer's idea is to give students cards and ask them to write a few lines expressing a personal opinion on the issues. The cards are collected and redistributed so that no one knows whose card they are holding. Then students are asked to read that card aloud and take a minute to agree or disagree. In this way, the issue is aired, diversity exposed, the unspeakable spoken, and a foundation for real conversation laid. This brings me to the notion of generating dialogue rather than discussion.

☐   Generate dialogue

Many authors have argued that dialogue is preferable to discussion in generating critical thinking and new insights (Daft, 2007; Freire, 1972; Senge, 1994), as discussion merely achieves the statement of position and can meander without direction, whereas dialogue can reveal feelings and explore assumptions such that common ground and shared meanings are built. Yet discussion is the way most people communicate. It is also a common aim in lesson plans.

In the transformative classroom, however, communication works best when it is used with conscious intent. Discussion can be transformed into dialogue by establishing three conditions: learners try to suspend their assumptions, learners see each other as equal team members, and a facilitator is there to ensure that everyone has a chance to contribute.

☐   Rethink assessment: Produce tangible products of that voice

For voice and dialogue to have meaning, it is useful, indeed important, to set assessment and other learning activities that have a purpose larger than the mere testing of knowledge. Good assessment actually serves two purposes: it provides an opportunity to provide guidance and feedback to the learner; and it provides a means to ensure that minimum standards of entry to a profession are maintained. Essays, clinical reports, journals, posters and tutorial presentations and other commonly used assessment items remain useful in the transformative context, especially when they are designed to (i) directly contribute to the professional/social world, (ii) be personally engaging, and (iii) stimulate reflection.

Table 11.2 Examples of critical thinking assessment converted into constructive thinking activities

Critical thinking topics	Constructive thinking topics
Conduct a client interview and provide a report documenting your psychosocial assessment skills.	Conduct a client interview and provide a summary documenting your psychosocial assessment skills, and then find a classmate who will provide an appraisal of your strengths and areas for improvement.
In a 2000-word essay, critically analyse how risk management takes place in a relevant public health facility.	After critically reflecting on risk management processes in a relevant public health facility, create a flyer/brochure to inform consumers and carers.
Visit a consulting room in your local health service in your role as an ordinary citizen. Using the literature on waiting, engagement and anxiety reduction, critique the experience.	Using your knowledge of waiting rooms, engagement and anxiety reduction, describe an ideal consulting room setting providing a justification for the decisions that you make.

In my experience, assessment items are not usually designed in these ways and as a result the activity may promote critical thinking, but not necessarily add anything to the social world. It isn't difficult, though, to make small changes to conventional assessment items to deepen the learner's constructive thinking. Taylor (2007, p. 182) calls this 'creating artefacts of mind' – that is, setting activities that produce tangible products wherein ideas that stem from the learning experience are made available for others (see Table 11.2 for examples where critical thinking assessment items are converted into constructive activities).

The assessment thus becomes a social communication activity and a potential change project. In this way assessment activities, like the student–teacher relationship, contributes to the transformational experience.

■ Conclusion

This chapter has provided a rationale for a viable alternative to the transmission mode of teaching that unfortunately remains the prevailing model of teaching in many academic settings and one where communication flows from the expert teacher to the receiving student. The transformational model operates differently by emphasising transaction, places the lens of enquiry squarely onto issues of inequity and marginalisation, emphasises the need for change not just understanding, and argues that whilst technical skills need to be practised, so too does the language of possibility, for it is here that constructive ideas for the future will emerge.

References

Baumgartner, L. (2002). Living and learning with HIV/AIDS: Transformational tales continued. *Adult Education Quarterly, 53*, 44–70.

Conway, J. (2001). *A Woman's Education.* Toronto: Knopf.

Cragg, C., Plotnikoff, R., Hugo, K. and Casey, A. (2001). Perspective transformation in RN-to-BSN distance education. *Journal of Nursing Education, 40*, 317–322.

Daft, R. (2007). *The Leadership Experience (4th ed.)* Hampshire: Thomson.

Dickinson, E. (1960). The gleam of an heroic act. In T.H. Johnson (ed.) *The Complete Poems.* Boston: Little Brown.

Feinstein, B. (2004). Learning and transformation in the context of Hawaiian traditional ecological knowledge. *Adult Education Quarterly, 54*, 105–120.

Freire, P. (1972). *Pedagogy of the Oppressed.* Harmondsworth: Penguin.

Gee, J. and Lankshear, C. (1995). The new work order: Critical language awareness and 'Fast Capitalism' Texts. *Discourse: Studies in the Cultural Politics of Education, 16*, 5–19.

Giroux, H. (2000). *Impure Acts: The Practical Politics of Cultural Studies.* New York: Routledge.

Goldie, J., Schwartz, L. and Morrison, J. (2005). Whose information is it anyway? Informing a 12-year patient of her terminal prognosis. *Journal of Medical Ethics, 31*, 427–434.

Greene, M. (1995). Art and imagination: Overcoming a desperate stasis. *Phi Delta Kappan, 76*(1), 378–382.

Greene, M. (1995). *Releasing the Imagination: Essays on Education, the Arts, and Social Change.* San Francisco: Jossey-Bass.

Habermas, J. (1972). *Knowledge and Human Interests.* (trans. J. Shapiro). London: Heinemann.

Herrera, H. (1991). *The Little Deer by Frida Kahlo: The Paintings.* London: Bloomsbury, p. 189.

Hobbs, R. and Frost, R. (2003). Measuring the acquisition of media-literacy skills. *Reading Research Quarterly, 38*, 330–355.

King, K. (2000). The adult ESL experience: Facilitating perspective transformation in the classroom. *Adult Basic Education, 10*, 69–89.

Luthar, S. (2003). *Resilience and Vulnerability: Adaptation in the Context of Childhood Adversities.* New York: Columbia University.

Lyon, D. (2001). *Surveillance society Monitoring everyday life.* Open University Press, Buckingham.

MacLeod, R. D., Parkins, C., Pullon, S. and Robertson, G. (2003). Early clinical exposure to people who are dying: Learning to care at the end of life. *Medical Education, 37*(1), 51–58.

McAllister, M. (2005). Transformative teaching in nursing education: Preparing for the Possible. *Collegian, 12*(1), 13–18.

McAllister, M., Tower, M., and Walker, R. (2007). Gentle interruptions: Transformative approaches to clinical teaching. *Journal of Nurse Education, 46*(7), 304–312.

McAllister, M. and Rowe, J. (2003). Blackbirds singing in the dead of night? Advancing dialogue on the craft of teaching qualitative health research. *Journal of Nursing Education, 42*(7), 296–303.

Mezirow, J. (1991). *Transformative Dimensions of Adult Learning.* San Francisco, CA: Jossey-Bass.

Mezirow, J. (2000). *Learning as Transformation.* San Francisco: Jossey-Bass.

O'Sullivan, E. and Morrell, A., eds. (2002). *Expanding the Boundaries of Transformative Learning: Essays on Theory and Praxis.* New York: Palgrave Press, p. 18.

Palmer, P. (1998). *The Courage to Teach.* San Francisco: Jossey Bass.

Quin, R. and McMahon, B. (1991). *Media Analysis: Performance in Media in Western Australian Government Schools* (excerpted for Media Literacy Review, Media Literacy Online Project, College of Education) Oregon: University of Oregon. Accessed on the Internet on 26/09/07 at http://interact.uoregon.edu/MediaLit/mlr?readings/articles/standard.html.

Ralston, Saul, J. (2005). *The Collapse of Globalism: And the Reinvention of the World.* Toronto: Penguin.

Senge, P. (1994). *The Fifth Discipline: The Art & Practice of the Learning Organization.* New York: DoubleDay.

Taylor, E. (2007). An update of transformative learning theory: A critical review of the empirical research (1999–2005). *International Journal of Lifelong Learning. 26*(2), 173–191.

Thayer-Bacon, B. (2000). *Transforming Critical Thinking: Thinking Constructively.* New York: Teachers College Press.

Part 3

Education Beyond the Classroom for Health and Social Care

Part 3 brings the book's exploration to a close with five chapters that look at how health and social care professionals have an opportunity to shape their own futures and what might influence these processes. In Part 2 of the book, recognising that sometimes the familiar can be a valuable resource in promoting learning was explored. In Chapter 12, Maureen Deacon provides an example of this approach being used not only in terms of teaching and learning, but in promoting opportunities for more effectively understanding the nuances and values inherent in everyday practice. She successfully makes the familiar strange in her ethnographic account of work she was involved in Acute Mental Health Care. Interestingly, this is an area of health and social care that has endured many staffing difficulties, in terms of both recruitment and retention. As the nature of health and social care moves ever further away from what has been seen to be familiar and traditional, preparing, recruiting and retaining staff will become an important issue. In Chapter 13, Dawn Freshwater and Philip Esterhuizen provide a stimulating challenge to how such issues may be tackled by the way in which we value and work with each other from the early days of training to becoming an experienced practitioner. An insightful analysis of the concepts of love, relationships and the harsh realities of practice is presented.

In Chapter 14, drawing on an equally large canvas, Naomi Sharples explores the difficulties and challenges in making education for health and social care accessible to all. Drawing upon her work with deaf people, both in practice and in education, a thought-provoking account is presented of the notion of marginalised groups and how such individuals are often excluded in a society that seeks perfection in all things. Reporting on her pioneering and innovative work in this area, an alternative range of possibilities are revealed. Whilst clear challenges to many traditional health and social care institutions and organisations are identified, ways forward in

171

responding to these are presented. The penultimate chapter, Chapter 15, in Part 3 takes the reader back to what for many readers was the start of their own careers in health and social care. Mike Hazelton, Rachel Rossiter and Ellen Sinclair report on the work they have been doing in preparing those qualified students to become confident and capable practitioners in their early days of learning to become a health and social care professional.

The final account in Part 3 and the book is an End Note presented by Tony Warne and Sue McAndrew. The prevailing themes that have emerged in the construction and development of this book are teased out and assembled for the reader.

Chapter 12

'Going native' in the inner city: Learning about caring by promoting and utilising practice-based evidence

Maureen Deacon

■ Introduction

This chapter explores the educational importance of learning from real-life practice, and suggests ways to achieve this routinely and creatively. These activities can be used in both classroom and practice settings. The importance of learning from real-life practice is often misunderstood or remains unrecognised. Conscious deliberation of, and accountable learning from, routine and real-life practice can provide important and challenging learning opportunities. Garfinkel (1967), in his seminal text, argued that not only do experts find it hard to examine what they routinely do, they actually find it strange and sometimes even irritating when this is asked of them. To an expert such matters are 'blindingly obvious' and this can be explained by the notion of being 'unconsciously competent'.

Take, for example, a familiar situation found in many areas of health and social care – how the care of individuals is organised? In hospital wards, for example, the ward office will often contain the ubiquitous white dry wipe board. These are usually a significant tool for organising and managing how patients' needs are to be met (so might contain information about diagnosis and treatment) and also they can be used for the organisation of the staff working in that area. Sometimes they indicate to whom a patient 'belongs' (consultant name). These different kinds of information are attended to in multiple ways. I can remember one day asking two nurses to explain their use of such a whiteboard to me. They were amused and a little bewildered by my interest. They struggled to articulate how they used their board, and the conversation ended with the comment 'well, they're the heart and lungs of the ward really'.

I found it interesting that here was a bundle of work activities (Hughes, 1971), evidently of vital importance, yet these nurses struggled to explain this work. Here I am not criticising – they were expert nurses going about their routine business and getting their work done. Indeed it could be argued that the routinism of work is an essential component of organisational life. Not much would get done if practitioners had to constantly and carefully consider their every manoeuvre in great detail and depth. However, if routine work is mostly what practitioners do, then it is crucial that it is examined for three reasons:

(1) Individuals will mostly experience the routine practice of health and social care practitioners by being in receipt of routine care, whilst improved patient care is the object of practice development.

(2) In order to systematically and creatively develop practice it is imperative that we look at what practitioners spend most of their time doing. Anything else is merely the 'icing on the cake'.

(3) Effective practice development begins with rigorous examination of where we are now and moves on from this to analysing where it is practically possible to go next.

One approach for encouraging health and social care students to think about and explore the routines inherent in their everyday practice would be through utilising the research process. Whilst most programmes of learning delivered in higher education incorporate the promotion of research, for many students these are often experienced as complex processes that cannot always be conceptualised as having a relationship to their everyday practice. However, perhaps by encouraging students to use research approaches to explore specific aspects of their practice, bringing their 'findings' back to the university for analysis, synthesis and explication of meaning, the research agenda may become a more integrated aspect of their future practice.

In exploring the above three issues I intend to demonstrate how an ethnographic approach can be used to explicate some of the complexities inherent in everyday practice. I will draw upon my work with people who are acutely mentally ill, and who because of their illness often require treatment in an in-patient setting. Like all contemporary care settings, mental health care is multi-professional and aims to provide integrated health and social care. Given my background is nursing, the examples I draw upon are inevitably concerned with the work of nurses. However, I argue that my analysis of the opportunities to learn from the routine experience of practice can be applied in other health and social care contexts.

■ Developing an ethnographic approach

The methods involved in ethnographic study can provide many useful strategies for learning from practice and this is discussed below. Much has been written about learning from practice. One genre has involved the application of general educational theory to practice and such theories are multifarious, including humanist and behavioural approaches (Canham and Moore, 2002). More contemporary approaches have included the promotion of clinical supervision (Gilmore, 2001), reflective practice (Johns, 2006) and critical thinking (Jones-Devitt and Smith, 2007). Whilst these different methods have many family resemblances, there is a tendency to see these approaches as somehow being disembodied from the everyday work of the health and social care practitioners. Supervision, for example, is concerned with the explication of the interpersonal relationship between practitioner and patient/client, potentially, leading to the improvement of practice. However, despite this being widely understood and recognised, it is often a missing element of everyday and routine practice, being reserved to those discrete and particular therapeutic encounters. Thus the idea of reflection *in* action (Schon, 1983) is often reduced to the 'coffee break debrief'.

Arguably what is required is the raising of awareness of the learning that can be gained by the anthropological concept of trying to 'make the familiar strange' (Pollner and Emerson, 2001). This is a strategy often employed by ethnographer and those interested in hearing other people's stories (see also Barker and Buchanan-Barker's comments in Chapter 3). Importantly, such an approach has the potential to open up practice for scrutiny and provides an important condition for ensuring accountability in action.

Unlike many early anthropologists, contemporary practitioners working within a familiar setting do not need to 'go native'. The challenge is to learn from what is largely taken for granted and this demands particular skills from practitioners. For example, a need to persistently ask questions about routine practices, to try to get into another's shoes by creatively considering the practice scene from an alternative perspective, or to disrupt the routine by doing mundane things differently. The latter has the potential to be a more risky strategy. Whilst each of these approaches requires a degree of confidence, particularly when it comes to handling organisational politics, as educationalists, these are activities we should be encouraging amongst students who are exposed to practice-based learning as part of their studies.

To ask questions about routine matters means that you have to notice what they are. A good place to start is by looking at the big organisational picture: what goes on when and how is the organisation's routine temporally structured? What are the practical implications of this routine for the different stakeholders in this setting and whose interests are being served by it?

For example, in the context of responding to a child thought to be at risk, the child's case conference is usually a multi-professional and multi-agency affair that will systematically explore a range of evidence before considering a particular course of action. Applying 'the making the familiar strange' approach to the examination of such meetings is likely to reveal the highly complex activity involved and the practical consequences for different individuals in terms of future work or outcomes. Often such complexities reflect the unconscious playing out of professional socialisation, which will in turn impact on the interpersonal relationship between professionals (Stark et al., 2002).

An alternative approach in making the familiar strange is that of 'imagining' (Morgan, 1984); for example, imagining what would matter most if, as a patient, you were admitted to hospital for emergency treatment. In this situation, whilst the environment cues are familiar (the bed, curtains and so on), the context is unfamiliar and likely to be frightening, distressing and full of uncertainty. As a patient, it might be that the 'routine' skills of a kind, person-centred, calm practitioner might be more important than the technical interventions available. Likewise, being subjected to 'routine observation' in this situation could feel either intrusive or reassuring or both simultaneously.

Another example might be to think of yourself in another role such as social worker. How might you feel in attending a client review meeting where it is felt to be important to provide your client with services they need, but knowing that there is a long waiting list for such services.

These creative imaginings can lead us to new questions: what is the purpose of this activity? Is there a better way to do it? If we did it this way rather than that way what would be the advantages and disadvantages and so on? Answering such questions is part of the ethnographic approach to enquiry and learning. An ethnographic approach is concerned with analysing how parts of a particular social world are connected to its whole. The research method most closely associated with ethnography is participant-observation, whereby the researcher takes part in the social group being studied. This advantages the researcher by giving them close access to the social group and particularly to their interpretive context; that is, the ways in which they constantly give their social world meaning.

However, Garfinkel and Wieder (1992) note that in order to rigorously research a social group the researcher must have sufficient expertise to be able to interpret the particular case under examination. This facilitates an approach that avoids asking 'why aren't these nurses doing x, y and z?' to one that asks 'what are they doing, how are they doing it and why are they doing it this way?'

This is a critically important difference because it leads to an insider, rather than outsider perspective, and this, along with understanding its practice as a 'method of discovery' (Fielding, 1993: 155), is the hallmark of ethnography.

■ Using an ethnographic approach

Using an ethnographic approach allows us to examine social action in context. For example, it draws our attention to the fact that at any one point in time, the practice of health and social care is likely to be both constrained and/or enhanced by a range of organisational imperatives. Often health and social care professionals need to become 'multi-taskers' and experts in handling multiple realities, multiple needs and multiple demands. This is accomplished by endless, open-ended, diffuse and contingent activities whereby new work has to be constantly added in and woven into ongoing work.

Getting to grips with what the organisational imperatives are in any particular environment can be a challenge but, as they provide the interpretive context for formulating the work to be done, it can be a very useful learning strategy. Some purchase can be gained through the following activities:

- Pick a routine activity and explain in detail how it is done and why it is done that way.
- Observe for common phrases used by practitioners in the setting and unpack their meaning and evidence base.
- Imagine that you have to explain a piece of mundane action to an alien visiting Earth for the first time.
- Consider how a service user would answer the question 'Given your experience of this service, what do you think is the most important thing to the professionals involved?'

In the context of the case used here (the acute in-patient mental health unit) for exploring this ethnographic approach, the organisational imperatives were revealed to coalesce around: discharging patients as quickly as possible; preventing patients' disturbance from exposing the organisation to criticism; accomplishing this by following rules and by fitting in with the wider organisation and other agencies. Thus to understand the work of a specific group of health and social care professionals we have to understand the organisational context in which they do that work. Not always easy to do. For example, Dingwall and Allen (2001) argued that within nursing the activity between nurses and individual patients has largely been regarded as the central site of interest when considering practice development; yet in reality, it is the organisational context of practice that has the most influence on the work that is done. In setting the scene for the example of learning about how to care for disturbed patients, such realities are clearly visible.

■ Deconstructing disturbance

Caring for disturbed patients was necessary on the acute ward because they were too ill for formal therapy and community care. Indeed it was the patients' level of disturbance that had brought them into hospital in the first place. However, the imperative to contain patients' disturbance was predominantly nurses' work and in this context probably the most challenging aspect of the nurses' work and is occupationally unique (May and Kelly, 1982).The process of effectively caring for people who were acutely disturbed promoted the necessary conditions for treatment whereby a person could be restored to a state of social equilibrium when they could potentially benefit from ongoing therapeutic interventions.

Patients who are disturbed can also be disturbing to others (Barker, 2003; Winship, 1995); for example, a lady with early onset dementia who is admitted to a medical ward for physical health problems. It can be upsetting to be with people who are extremely distressed. It can be frightening to be with someone who is hostile, threatening and potentially violent. It can be irritating to be with someone who asks you the same question over and over again. It can be infuriating when someone follows the same course of action that has led them predictably into trouble on repeated occasions. It can be alarming when people do strange things that you cannot comprehend. Patients then can disturb each other, their family and friends and those caring for them.

'Disturbance' as a glossing device is useful to nurses. It indicates a situated level of severity – thus a patient's progress can be measured on a scale of 'more or less disturbed'. It also provides an assessment of the type of nursing work that the patient requires: a 'horrible and disturbed' patient like Stan had to be steered away from other patients, particularly another disturbed and hostile patient, for his protection. A *disturbed and terrified* patient like Katherine needed to be tenderly comforted and protected from others.

It was this disturbance and its social consequences that brought people to the acute ward and the most disturbed to the psychiatric intensive care unit (PICU). Locating notions of disturbance within constructs of mental illness enables the nurse to know *how* to attribute meaning and to know *what* to practically do about social matters out of place. The latter describes social actions that in some circumstances might be considered quite normal and socially acceptable but out of context become signs of mental illness. For example, a patient's high level of sexual arousal and subsequent desire to engage in frequent sexual relations might be conceptualised as a sign of their mental illness from which they require protection. In other contexts they might be judged promiscuous, or as a person who simply enjoys sex.

Concepts of mental illness were used by the nurses as resources for explaining and managing social matters out of place. But judging a patient's level of responsibility for their actions is never an entirely settled matter because it has to be situated in each and every case on each and every occasion that is required for different practical purposes. Both May and Kelly (1982) and Bowers (1995) have noted that rather than being a 'black and white' issue, questions of absolution are indexical matters as much answered for utilitarian reasons as judgements based on evidence.

Thus, caring for people who are in crisis has to be achieved within the context of attempting to meet the organisational imperatives. Often the organisational context does not allow for alternative approaches whereby patients can be kept safe whilst they receive a service focused on their growth and development (Huxley, 2000). Additionally, due to the intensity of many acute mental health settings, the majority of the patients are acutely disturbed to a greater or lesser extent. Devoting lots of attention to some disturbed patients inevitably means devoting less attention to others and this is a continuing trouble for nurses (Deacon, 2003). Just how much share would an individual patient get of a nurse's skilled attention is entirely contingent on the care of all the other patients and the broader organisational circumstances.

The nurses' management of acute disturbance is embedded in their development of a 'natural attitude'. The idea that mental health nurses use *themselves* as therapeutic agents have been a topic of much interest (see Gallop, 1997; Speedy, 1999). Growing interest among nurses in the use of technical 'tools' such as activity schedule recording (Baguley and Baguley, 2002) and rating scales for assessing psychotic symptoms (Siddle and Everitt, 2002) is usually presented with the caveat that they are used within the context of a therapeutic relationship. Health and social care professionals are encouraged to work respectfully, optimistically, collaboratively and empathically with their patients (Repper, 2002).

However, the nurses on the acute ward often have to work with patients who are unable to straightforwardly engage with them in such ways. Like many professionals they are often faced with patients who are hostile, irritable, labile and over-familiar. Many are so 'ill' that they have little sense of the needs of anybody else and can be completely absorbed with their own preoccupations to the detriment of others. Occasionally, some patients are threatening, some are violent and some are extremely demanding. Some patients are isolative and discourage all attempts to engage with staff. Some talk incomprehensibly and some about topics considered the products of delusions. It is for these reasons that patients are considered too ill for therapy. Paradoxically, a patient's ability to begin to engage in therapeutic relationships and talk as a competent individual is seen as a sign of improvement and a harbinger of discharge from the ward.

Unlike the case in the acute ward, the 'problem' patient on a surgical ward stands out from the crowd because such behaviour is unexpected and abnormal. Caring for disturbed patients is the *raison d'être* of nurses working in acute mental health care services, and where they *expect* their patients to be disturbed and difficult to care for. This, after all, is why people are admitted to the unit. Distinctions lie more in questions about *just* how disturbed and *just* how difficult particular patients are.

Directly engaging with patients' disturbance involved efforts to treat its perceived causes and to ameliorate its social outcomes. The former was achieved in the majority of cases by treatment with drugs. In keeping with general psychiatric practice (Okocha, 2001), drug treatment was the mainstay of biomedical endeavour in the acute unit. As in many other situations, facilitating the patients' return to a state of equilibrium was achieved primarily through drug therapy.

The other main method of direct engagement was interactional. Using talk and activity, nurses attempted to develop with patients a less disturbing version of reality. All formal 'talking therapies' work from the premise that reality construction is an interactional activity but, as discussed earlier, the majority of patients in the acute unit were too ill for such therapy. Here this interactional activity was often of short duration and had a specific focus. It often involved problem-solving, comforting and confrontation. Problem-solving was initiated by a patient's complaint.

The nurse would listen carefully to what the patient was saying, interpret it, reporting back their interpretation and attempt to negotiate a solution. This tactic could take variable amounts of time. For example, I recall a patient coming into the office one time. She sat down looking very distressed and dishevelled and began an agitated, convoluted story addressed to Bill (a Charge Nurse) that I found very hard to follow. Bill listened hard, asked her to explain several things again and clarified certain points to check out his understanding. He asked her calmly to slow down and try to talk more quietly so that he could better understand her. He gradually interpreted that she was worried about the security of her flat and did not know where her keys were. Eventually they agreed that he would attempt to contact her neighbour and ascertain whether or not her flat was secure.

Comforting patients was accomplished by listening, reassurance and physical contact. Late one night, an older patient, Agnes, was literally 'tucked into bed' by a nursing assistant. Agnes was agitated, disorganised and distressed. She moaned loudly and frequently and made comments that irritated the other patients to the extent that she was told to 'get lost' by another patient. She was very upset, saying that this event had reminded her of how her family 'didn't want her either'. The nursing assistant dried her tears, reassured her that it would all be forgotten by the morning, helped her prepare for bed, tucked her in and turned off the lights.

Nurses confronted patients who were disturbed when they became too anti-social. This usually meant that they were threatening the safety of the ward environment or disturbing its peace. Despite being mentally ill, some matters could not be 'let go'. Sophie, for example, was 'told off' for going on leave and returning to the ward late at night, drunk, truculent and noisy. This, she was told when she had sobered up the next morning, was extremely unfair to other patients who were ill and needed their sleep.

Rarely, direct engagement involved physical restraint of patients by nurses. This was observed when a recently admitted patient suddenly, without apparent warning, became threatening and violent in the lounge area of the ward. Sue and I were asked to clear the area of other patients and visitors. Having accomplished this, we stood at the doors to the lounge in order to prevent anybody going in again. Sue, having recently qualified, told me that this was the aspect of the work that she liked least and dreaded most. She recounted a tale concerning a similar experience. On this occasion, she said, she had afterwards been approached by a visitor who had complimented her on her work. The visitor had marvelled over the difficulties of the job and reflected that he would be unable to do it. As Emerson and Pollner (1975) note, judging the moral worth of work is in the perspective of the judger, rather than being intrinsic to the activity. Sue reported that she had been really taken aback by this but that the encounter had made her think afresh about restraint.

The strategy of direct engagement in the management of acute disturbance/crisis included some of the 'dirty work' of the occupation. The natural attitude of the nurses, resting as it does on the artful exoneration of anti-social behaviour, is a 'dignifying rationalization' (Hughes, 1971: 340) that alleviates both the mundane and the unusual unpleasantness of the work. Such dirty work, amongst other things, might be avoided by the use of trouble avoidance strategies.

For example, surveillance (keeping patients under constant watch) is a trouble avoidance strategy through which they could meet the organisational imperatives. 'Anticipating trouble' practices are also located in individual matters and individual patient's cases, often being so mundane that it is hard to notice them. On just one occasion I managed to study the PICU team's patient review process. During this I observed Mike (a Staff Nurse) skilfully synchronising a complex social event that involved patients, their families, professional staff and students. Mike competently coordinated a whole sequence of practical matters. Towards the end of the meeting it was stated that it was now John's turn to be discussed. This patient's name had cropped up in an earlier discussion regarding another patient called Mani. Mike had reported that John intimidated Mani and this information had added to the team's determination to treat Mani effectively and move him on from the PICU. Now it was John's turn to be considered, and the staff nurse started preparations for what he called 'damage limitation'. He reported that John was keen to come and talk with the team – he wanted to negotiate some leave. The tray of drinks was removed along with stray cups and Mike asked the students (and me) to leave the room. He explained that during the review meeting in the previous week, John had become threatening and aggressive when his requests were not met. The tray of drinks had been smashed and used as a weapon.

Trouble avoidance strategies were also employed in relation to the difficulties of patients living together. Calming down arguments and breaking up fights between patients – peacekeeping – was nursing work. Some social matters out of place were ignored. Others were minimised through techniques of distraction, through humour, postponement and comforting interactions, and through non-verbal signs of disapproval. The degree to which the matter was considered to be anti-social was related to the choice of technique. The strategy of minimising strangeness served the purpose of containing the consequences of patients' disturbance whilst their mental illness was treated.

These methods of dealing with difficult situations have been established by carefully and systematically learning from practice and by 'making the familiar strange', and it is to these topics that I now return.

■ Learning from ethnography

I have used a particular case to illuminate how the ethnographic approach can help us learn from practice and below I offer an exercise to enable this learning method to be used in any setting. It can be done alone but will be more effective in a group workshop format (because this interactional process encourages accountability).

- Describe the activity that you spent most time on when you were last at work.
- Explain the factors that you had to consider in choosing how to go about that activity – try and include as many as possible.
- Discuss how the activity contributed to the organisation's goals.
- Consider one small change that might improve the effectiveness of the activity.
- Explain exactly how you would go about making this change and predict some of the troubles that might emerge and how you can prevent them.

Health and social care professionals working within a familiar setting clearly do not need to go native – they are already deeply native. Their challenge is to learn from what they largely take for granted by making the familiar strange and this demands particular skills from practitioners. These can be conceptualised as accountability in action.

To be accountable means to answer for our actions and to take full responsibility for those actions. For nurses and other health and social care professionals this is the critical nub of professional practice. To be personally accountable requires that we know what we are doing and why we are doing it and that we can be able to explain this. It does not mean taking responsibility for an imperfect world but it does mean taking responsibility for how we act within that imperfect world. It follows that in order to know what we are doing we need to be able to examine and articulate our practice (Deacon et al., 2006). Accountable practitioners, at times, have to deliberately bypass their 'unconscious competence' in order to do this. This requires practitioners to be conscientiously committed to developing their practice, to be confident enough to open up their practice to careful scrutiny and to be prepared to change what they do if necessary. Contemporaneously, these strategies are often glossed by the idea of the reflective practitioner, though Fook et al. (2006) note that this too runs the risk of becoming mechanical and ill-considered in the context of its enduring popularity.

Accountable practitioners have the responsibility for facilitating the learning of others. Whilst positive role-modelling of doing the work is a highly effective educational strategy (Donaldson and Carter, 2005), concurrently explaining it and sharing critical reflection on it is, arguably, the gold standard (though, of course, not always practically possible). However, if practitioners cannot explain what they do and why they do it, then this gold standard of education in practice is unachievable. They have to robustly own their work and this includes confronting positively the stigma and shame of what some may consider its unattractive, 'dirty' aspects.

Routine things can be done differently in small but practice-changing ways. Understanding nursing work differently enables us to see more realistically its therapeutic value. For example, I observed how a nurse helping a patient do his laundry had multiple purposes beyond the most obvious of getting his laundry done. How the patient was during this activity became a taken-for-granted document of his current mental state and its comparison to his past and future mental state. This, in turn, became part of the bigger story of his recovery and how to enable it. In conducting the activity with him the nurse therapeutically managed his acute irritability, labile mood and suspiciousness by effectively using the methods of caring for a disturbed patient. She also promoted his social inclusion by improving upon his dishevelled and malodorous state. Later I heard another nurse complimenting him on his smartness. The patient rewarded him with a big smile rather than the usual irritable and suspicious response. Articulating this practice rather than ignoring it as too unimportant to even consider is a method for practice development that can be attended to routinely. Even if just once a week a mundane piece of professional work is unpicked like this the opportunities to improve that aspect of practice are creatively revealed. In addition, bigger questions can be asked as practitioners '... develop the capacity to resist and transgress' (Fook et al., 2006) for the purpose of improving the organisational context of care.

■ Conclusion

In summary, this chapter has argued that learning from practice is an essential component of its development. Qualitative research methods such as ethnography can provide a systematic framework for explicating and harnessing these important insights into practice. However, aspects of these methods also promise routine practice development techniques, which, in turn, can bring research to life and demystify it. All students can be directed to these methodologies via encouraging them in the classroom to explore how *they* make sense of practice (by observation, by noticing the everyday organisational discourses, by participating in the team's work, by listening to patient's stories, etc.) and helping to transpose those sense-making activities to theoretical and philosophical models of research.

For the student of practice, learning from the real world of health and social care results, for the successful, in becoming an organisational native. This is a desirable state given that organisations need employees who can competently get on with the work at hand and given that practitioners need to be confident about their work activities. However, it is simultaneously undesirable because it can lead to organisational blindness, trap us in practices that do not best serve the needs of those using them and, at worst, lead to complacency. Systematically and conscientiously learning from practice allows practitioners to engage with the tensions involved in going native. This is not always a comfortable position but few enter the helping professions expecting it to be an easy life.

References

Baguley, I. and Baguley, C. (2002) Psychological treatment for anxiety and depression in schizophrenia. In: Harris, N., Williams, S. and Bradshaw, T. (Eds) *Psychosocial Interventions for People with Schizophrenia. A Practical Guide for Mental Health Workers.* Basingstoke: Palgrave MacMillan.

Barker, P. (2003) Putting acute care in its place. *Mental Health Nursing*, 23 (1), 12–15.

Bowers, L. (1995) *Mental Illness as a Social Phenomenon.* PhD Thesis. Manchester: The University of Manchester.

Canham, J. and Moore, S. (2002) Learning approaches in the practice context. In: Canham, J. and Bennet, J. (Eds) *Mentorship in Community Nursing: Challenges and Opportunities.* London: Blackwell Science.

Deacon, M. (2003) Caring for people in the 'virtual ward': The practical ramifications for acute nursing work. *Journal of Psychiatric and Mental Health Nursing*, 10 (4), 465–471.

Deacon, M., Warne, T. and McAndrew, S. (2006) Closeness, chaos and crisis: The attractions of working in acute mental health care. *Journal of Psychiatric and Mental Health Nursing*, 13, 750–757.

Dingwall, R. and Allen, D. (2001) The implications of healthcare reforms for the profession of nursing. *Nursing Inquiry*, 8 (2), 64–74.

Donaldson, J.H. and Carter, D. (2005) The value of role modelling: Perceptions of undergraduate and diploma (adult) students. *Nurse Education in Practice*, 5, 353–359.

Emerson, R.M. and Pollner, M. (1975) Dirty work designations: Their features and consequences in a psychiatric setting. *Social Problems*, 23, 243–254.

Fielding, N. (1993) Ethnography. In: Gilbert, N. (Ed.) *Researching Social Life.* London: Sage Publications.

Fook, J., White, S. and Gardner, F. (2006) Critical reflection: A review of contemporary literature and understandings. In: White, S., Fook, J. and Gardner, F. (Eds) *Critical Reflection in Health and Social Care*. Maidenhead: Open University Press.

Gallop, R. (1997) Caring about the client: The role of gender, empathy and power in the therapeutic process. In: Tilley, S. (Ed.) *The Mental Health Nurse. Views of Practice and Education*. Oxford: Blackwell Science.

Garfinkel, H. (1967) *Studies in Ethnomethodology*. Cambridge: Polity Press.

Garfinkel, H. and Wieder, L. (1992) Two incommensurable, asymmetrically alternate technologies of social analysis. In: Watson, G. and Seiler, R.M. (Eds) *Text in Context: Studies in Ethnomethodology*. London: Sage Publications.

Gilmore, A. (2001) Clinical supervision in nursing and health visiting: A review of the literature. In: Cutliffe, J.R., Butterworth, T. and Proctor, B. (Eds) *Fundamental Themes in Clinical Supervision*. London: Routledge.

Hughes, E.C. (1971) *The Sociological Eye: Selected Papers*. Chicago: Aldine.

Huxley, P. (2000) Alternatives to traditional mental health treatments. In: Newell, R. and Gournay, K. (Eds) *Mental Health Nursing, an Evidence-Based Approach*. London: Harcourt Publishers Ltd.

Johns, C. (2006) *Engaging Reflection in Practice: A Narrative Approach*, Oxford: Blackwell Publishing.

Jones-Devitt, S. and Smith, L. (2007) *Critical Thinking in Health and Social Care*. London: Sage Publications.

May, M.D. and Kelly, M.P. (1982) Chancers, pests and poor wee souls: Problems of legitimation in psychiatric nursing. *Sociology of Health and Illness*, 4, 279–297.

Morgan, J. (1984) "Le Misanthrop" and classical conceptions of character portrayal. *The Modern Language Review*, 79 (2), 290–300.

Okocha, C.I. (2001) Pharmacological therapy. In: Beer, M.D., Pereira, S.M. and Paton, C. (Eds) *Psychiatric Intensive Care*. London: Greenwich Medical Media Ltd.

Pollner, M. and Emerson, R.M. (2001) Ethnomethodology and ethnography. In: Atkinson, P., Coffey, A., Delamont, S., Lofland, J. and Lofland, L. (Eds) *Handbook of Ethnography*. London: Sage Publications.

Repper, J. (2002) The helping relationship. In: Harris, N., Williams, S. and Bradshaw, T. (Eds) *Psychosocial Interventions for People with Schizophrenia. A Practical Guide for Mental Health Workers*. Basingstoke: Palgrave MacMillan.

Schon, D.A. (1983) *The Reflective Practitioner. How Professionals Think in Action*. USA: Basic Books.

Siddle, R. and Everitt, J. (2002) Identifying and overcoming negative symptoms. In: Harris, N., Williams, S. and Bradshaw, T. (Eds) *Psychosocial Interventions for People with Schizophrenia. A Practical Guide for Mental Health Workers*. Basingstoke: Palgrave MacMillan.

Speedy, S. (1999) The therapeutic alliance. In: Clinton, M. and Nelson, S. (Eds) *Advanced Practice in Mental Health Nursing*. Oxford: Blackwell Science Ltd.

Stark, S., Stronach, I. and Warne, T. (2002) Teamwork in mental health: Rhetoric and reality. *Journal of Psychiatric and Mental Health Nursing*, 9, 411–418.

Winship, G. (1995) The unconscious impact of caring for acutely disturbed patients: A perspective for supervision. *Journal of Psychiatric and Mental Health Nursing*, 2, 227–231.

Chapter 13

Speaking the unspeakable: Emotional involvement

Dawn Freshwater and Philip Esterhuizen

■ Introduction

Love in various guises has been written about extensively. However, love in the modern idiom appears to have lost the romantic connotations of a bygone age and, as popular culture often suggests, has developed a brittleness and distance not generally associated with meaningful relationships. How does this apparent shift in values impact on those choosing a career in health and social care and what are the implications for educators and leaders? This chapter delves into this question using contemporary research into nursing socialisation to illustrate concepts affecting the ideals of those entering their chosen health and social care professions and the meaning of this for education and care delivery. We explore the underpinning context of the book: knowing me and understanding you; understanding this through the lens of self-awareness, reflective self-monitoring and self-interest, specifically in respect of the motivation to care and the development of therapeutic relationships. A search of the academic writings identifies little in terms of literature linking love and/or spirituality to health care professions, with the exception of nursing, counselling and psychotherapy. Although much of the literature underpinning this chapter is taken from these sources, our approach is generic and is intended to be transferable across and applicable to all health and social care professionals. Hence we develop a focus on the topical concept of attrition, and drawing on recent case studies, we highlight the emotional and psychological impact of an uncaring, caring, profession, asking, rather than answering, the question 'What's *has* love got to do with it?'

■ What is love anyway?

The extent of ancient manuscripts, books, songs and poetry dealing with and attempting to explain the mystery of human interaction is immeasurable. Many of these works deal with the eroticism and heroism of romantic interaction, rather than the underpinning interpersonal identification and connection (Freshwater and Robertson, 2002). This is an important distinction to make when entering a discourse on the notion of love within health and social care as any form of erotic attachment to the selfless and unconditional relationship between a health care professional and a patient/client is frowned upon and can carry a penalty from professional bodies, possible judicial consequences and social reproof from society in general. Indeed, as Watson (1998) observes, it is neither popular nor acceptable to speak of love in nursing circles. This reaction can be conceived as relating to the nature of the fiduciary relationship that health care professionals hold. That is to say that health care staff are perceived to be in a position of power in relation to the vulnerable patient/client (Esterhuizen, 1996). But the reaction can also be associated with the perception of the super-humanness of the health care professional; work with the most vulnerable in society has in the past been interpreted as a physical embodiment of spiritual ideals (see, for example, Watson, 1988; Taylor, 1994; Boykin & Schoenhofer, 2001; Stickley & Freshwater, 2002; Arman & Rehnsfeldt, 2006).

Suggestions of spiritual idealism are sure to spark a flurry of criticism – not least among groups of health care professionals themselves – that this interpretation is either a romanticised or an *ivory tower* philosophical discussion, not representing the reality of modern life. However, contemporary research has indicated that a spiritual approach to health care is a global phenomenon (Spence, 2001; Nåden & Eriksson, 2004; Esterhuizen, 2007; Callister & Freeborn, 2007; Maben et al., 2007).

Spirituality, in this discourse, should not be confused with religion although in some cultures the interpretation of unconditional love for one's fellow man has been influenced by Christianity, with Christian love and spirituality becoming synonymous with care and self-sacrifice (Dolan et al., 1983). Levinas discusses this confusion of love and spirituality (1991) with Christian values in society, and suggests that love, from a romanticised perspective, creates an interdependence: 'Love is the I satisfied by the thou, grasping in the other the justification of its being' (Levinas, 1991, p. 17); spirituality, on the other hand, being consciousness and truth (Levinas, 1991, p. 176). The idea of cultivating nurse–patient interdependency is against the ethos of supporting individuals to become independent and self-sufficient and smacks of dysfunctional behaviour. This distinction of erotic love as being destructive is highlighted by Stickley and Freshwater (2002), whereas ascetic, charitable love has the potential to be cleansing and transcendental. When seen from this perspective, perhaps the connotations of love in the current idiom as suggested at the start of this chapter are not that far removed from reality after all, but perhaps we shouldn't be speaking about *love* in caring, but rather about *spirituality;* with spirituality underpinning the concept of love.

Notwithstanding such qualifications and in the context of the previous debate we are still left with the question of how spirituality and/or love link with the notion of caring and education? In his research Nåden (2002) discusses the meeting between nurse and patient. He highlights the face-to-face encounter, drawing on work by Levinas (1991), in which, through having face-to-face contact, the responsibility for 'the other' is stressed. The I (self) sees the vulnerability in 'the Other' and the personal appeal for help seen in 'the Other's' face makes it morally unsound to refuse the call. This moral consciousness could equate to the love of self (I) and, by recognising the suffering of 'the Other', could therefore equate to the love of 'the Other'. It is this identification with one's own suffering, seen mirrored in the face of 'the Other', that allows us to care with compassion and unconditional regard – a phenomenon that some may call *love* (Freshwater & Robertson, 2002).

These findings by Nåden are echoed in Finch's research (Finch, 2006), which focused predominantly on nurse/patient communication. Indeed, Martin Buber (1958) elucidates clearly the distinction between an 'I–Thou' compassionate relationship and an 'I–It' objectifying relationship. The concept of compassion is in itself, however, not simply an emotional state, but is related to morality and the ethos of care (von Dietze & Orb, 2000) – a further complication to the notion of 'love'. While other authors have discussed Eros, agape and caritas, addressing the erotic, unselfish and charitable aspects of love (Watson, 1998; Stickley & Freshwater, 2002; Arman & Rehnsfeldt, 2006), the discussion in this chapter is framed by the practical notions of health and social care work and the perceptions of those involved in it.

■ Love and compassion in the workplace

Besides dealing with the challenges of a new role, dealing with patients is, in itself, a stressful situation for any new nursing student, but it is in working with patients that students learn to understand what it means to be a nurse in all its fullness. One might argue that it is through this work that the nurse begins not only to know the other, but also to know themselves. However basic and intrinsic to health care it may appear, students are, at first, afraid to actually work with patients. Their anxiety about making mistakes or (inadvertently) hurting patients is based in their moral approach to their new profession (Smith & Gray, 2001; Elliott, 2002), and being confronted by professional norms and values (often interpreted in specific ways by the various ward cultures) presents the student nurse with moral dilemmas (Randle, 2002; MacIntosh, 2003) and adds to the level of stress. Of course, some of the basic fear experienced also relates to the existential and neurotic aspects of being confronted with oneself (Freshwater & Robertson, 2002; Freshwater, 2000). The initially human response to 'doing good' emphasises the fact that nursing has, in essence, a moral base whether it is based on spirituality (Tanyi, 2002), personal reflection and reflexivity (Johns, 1998; Nåden & Eriksson, 2000), professional codes (Esterhuizen, 1996) or philosophical models (Widdershoven, 1999; Esterhuizen & Kooyman, 2001), although the distinction between these various approaches is not always clear and perhaps not even necessary.

Nursing is largely seen as being a practical profession, with a variety of skills forming the basis of the competencies being taught. As such, practice-based learning has a long history of being a powerful learning environment and beneficial to students. Consequently, responsibility for student preparation for patient contact falls on the nurse educationalist prior to the student entering the clinical arena. It is clear that experiential learning in the clinical area contains risks and limitations for both patient and student, but it does afford the opportunity to link theory to the realistic and lived world of caring. However, too little is done to develop the abstract skills students need, namely the various types of reflection, clinical decision-making or communication skills. A competency-based curriculum should address and assess abstract outcomes, taking into account the intent and emphasis of student learning (Johns, 2001).

There is another aspect of learning related to the practical aspects of nursing prior to the students being exposed to realities of the clinical setting. They need to be made aware of the myriad of variables contained in direct patient care. This could mean that part of the individual's objectives are assessed in terms of outcomes, whereas other aspects are more process-directed. In this instance, work by Driscoll (2000) can be beneficial and instrumental in supporting students to deconstruct their reality and formulate learning objectives (Figure 13.1).

The concept of wanting to 'do good' originates in the practicality of not wanting to cause unnecessary discomfort during procedures to wanting to 'do good' at a psychological, emotional or spiritual level. Nåden describes the interaction between a nurse and a patient, as she goes about her work without disturbing a patient lying with her eyes closed, and again interviews both parties. The nurse, aware that the patient needs rest, leaves her be, while the patient explains not feeling the need to please the nurse and, consequently, is able to focus on herself and meet her own needs for rest and relaxation. This, for the patient, means that she is able to use the energy she had conserved for the various therapies necessary to alleviate her illness (Nåden & Eriksson, 2000), and for doing things important to her well-being within the context of a hospital admission. It would appear that such *care* promotes caring for oneself, vital for both the health professional and the patient.

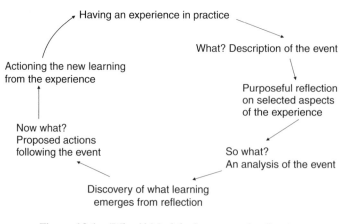

Figure 13.1 'What?' Model of structured reflection
Source: Driscoll (2000)

In trying to capture, and thus *teach*, the essence of such care, educators have attempted to incorporate service users in education and integrate their experience into the classroom experience for the student (see also Chapter 7). The rationale behind this approach is to narrow the gap between theory and practice settings and 'humanise' the patient population for the student, prior to entering the clinical field (Warne & McAndrew, 2004; Simons et al., 2006).

The patients in Nåden's research reported that they could 'feel' some nurses' presence without opening their eyes and just knew all was well. Van Manen, relating this to the concept of worry in his interesting and insightful scrutiny of worry as caring, seems to be speaking of a similar sort of presence that is intuitively experienced by the other. The concept of presence is not something that will be examined in detail here, however; it is, in our opinion pivotal to the effectiveness of the therapeutic relationship and indeed the student–teacher relationship. Suffice to say that, in our opinion, knowing self and other is a fundamental desire of all human beings and as such is a motivating factor in all human relations, impacting upon behaviours.

From an educational perspective, students could be stimulated to reflect on situations in which they feel satisfied that they dealt with the situation adequately. In this instance, use of a critical incident method or John's model for structured reflection could be appropriate (Johns, 2002). The rationale behind this approach is that they learn to (a) positively evaluate their successes, (b) identify skills, competencies and tactics that have worked for them and (c) recognise situations in which they are able to transfer their applied knowledge.

Reflection on successes, rather than shortcomings, can lead to an emancipated and self-confident awareness and so influence practice improvement (Driscoll, 2000; Becker Hentz & Lauterbach, 2005). Although the academic's 'core business' may be seen as education, it is important that personal development and professionalisation is not negated. While we can suggest all manner of teaching and learning sets, from an educational perspective emancipation and empowerment should be driving philosophical forces if stereotypical oppression within the hierarchy of health and social care is to be overturned (see also Chapters 1 and 2). From this perspective, educationalists need to be aware of the power they hold – 'thinking about thinking' has to be a principal ingredient of any empowering practice of education (Bruner, 1996, p. 19).

■ Example from practice: Motivation, predestination or calling?

In order to illustrate the embodiment and complexity of the motivation to care we highlight specific exemplars from Esterhuizen's research with Dutch student nurses based around five case studies (Esterhuizen, 2007). One of these concerns a student called Olga:

> She recounts how, one evening, she nursed a patient with a fractured ankle. This woman had fled Ghana, having seen her husband and children shot, and was awaiting a residence permit for the Netherlands. The woman appeared very sad and worked continually with her rosary. Regardless of being challenged by her colleagues on the ward, Olga followed her instinct that the patient needed to visit the hospital chapel. She felt that this activity formed a priority above the ward's evening routine and Olga was aware that, as a student, she ran the risk of reprimand in her assessment. The student described how, as she pushed the patient around the corner into the corridor leading to the chapel, they could see an almost life-size white marble statue of the Virgin Mary. On seeing the statue, the patient began to clap and sing and cry – an outpouring of emotion. Olga slowed before wheeling the patient into the main body of the chapel. Once inside, the patient again showed an emotional outpouring of (what appeared to be) grief and religious ecstasy. Olga's response to this situation was to 'do nothing', but was 'just with the patient'.

This resonates with work by Watson (1988), and Nåden and Eriksson (2000, 2002) on unconditionally 'being with' and is described in various forms in Freshwater (2002). Olga had no notions of these writings and so was not basing her responses on theoretical paradigms, but was following her intuition and what felt right to her. She was aware that the moment contained a certain spirituality and 'holiness' for the patient and she felt quite overcome by the situation – she was amazed at the 'warm feeling' it gave her. Although not formed by religious notions, having been brought up as an atheist by her parents, she found that she was rethinking what spirituality meant to her.

Reflecting on Levinas' work previously referred to, Olga's example seems to suggest that the recognition of another's suffering results directly in personal awareness and an attempt to understand the 'truth' of what it means. Although clear that she felt she was 'in the place' she needed to be, Olga maintained that hers was not specifically a philosophical reasoning or calling. Her response was based on her passion, interest and curiosity that she was now able to complement with her experience and increased insight. Olga's professional development appears to be occurring through an intrapersonal/transpersonal interaction; an important focus when considering caring as a philosophy (Nåden & Eriksson, 2002; Watson, 1988).

Reflecting on Olga's experience, one can imagine that it is difficult for the educationalist to artificially construct this calibre of reflective and learning situation routinely in a classroom setting, and unless personally experienced it will not make sense to other students and may well be inappropriate to use in other teaching situations. Role-play – as a stand-alone activity or as part of a workshop, whereby students enact situations calling for assertiveness, cultural competence or communication skills – is a cost-effective way of providing a 'safe' setting to experiment with new behaviour (Shearer & Davidhizar, 2003; Mc Cabe & Timmins, 2003; Ekebergh, Lepp & Dahlberg, 2004). However, educationalists should involve the student peer group to observe and provide feedback during the role-play, and ensure a thorough debriefing on conclusion. A retrospective assignment to incorporate the appropriate evidence-base could be a creative route to bridge the theory–practice divide and ensure applied student understanding of how to underpin abstract – and sometimes intuitive – concepts with literature and research.

This case study indicates that, in the 21st century in the Netherlands at least, in contrast to the seeming lack of attachment suggested in popular culture, students, by their own admission, were motivated to enter the caring professions by perceptions of a calling or predestination in some form or another.

What better explanation for motivation to enter a career in health care – to care for those vulnerable in society – than a feeling of calling or predestination? But it is more complex than this. In past years perceptions of the environment and the resulting influence they have on the individual have caused us to speculate that co-dependency could be a complicating factor in the health and social care professions. In a fairly dated but relevant exploratory study using the Friel Co-dependence Assessment Inventory and the modes of Roy's adaptation model, Chappelle and Sorrentino (1993) show that while 160 nurses showed responsibility, 65 showed varying degrees of co-dependent behavioural characteristics. Bennett, Robertson and Moss (1992) quote published co-dependency figures among nurses as ranging between 75% and 90%. They suggest that nursing serves, by virtue of its caring nature and its altruistic and ascetic origins, to attract those with a disposition to co-dependency (Malloy & Berkery, 1993; Yates & Mc Daniel, 1994; Gilmartin, 2000). This could be one explanation as to why the respondents in Esterhuizen's (2007) research perceived such a strong 'calling' to provide care, but to what degree are we in a position to pathologise an individual's beliefs and values (Esterhuizen, 2007)?

More recent literature questions the co-dependency statistics. Hopkins and Jackson (2002) and Martsolf (2002) suggest that this is not the case. Hopkins and Jackson (2002) found the incidence of co-dependent behaviour among nursing students no higher than among their contemporaries on other courses – they were, however, researching students and their learning in the academic setting and not in the hospital setting.

Whether students can or should be labelled as being co-dependent is not of particular importance. Health care educators should recognise the need to empower students to become more assertive and allow them to challenge the routines and rituals they encounter, as was the case in the situation Olga encountered. However, given that the majority of health care educators have themselves been socialised by and through the same processes, and may have similar motivations and drivers for entering the caring professions, we might also question the status of dependency and therein self–other boundaries within and across educational practices (see also Chapter 9).

Developing assertiveness, which is what we alluded to above, in and with students, can be seen as being positive, but not without risk (Freshwater, 1998). Espeland and Shanta (2001) discuss the dangers of dependency between student and faculty, while others (Philpin, 1999; Farrell, 2001; Randle, 2003) discuss the (student) nurse's dependency on colleagues in the clinical placement areas. According to Leyshon (2002), while seeking to break the status quo, educators do not actually provide the support students (or registered staff) need in re-establishing a new balance. This often leads to one authoritarian system being replaced by another.

■ Challenges to the individual's motivational calling

As in Olga's example, when confronted with the realities of work in the clinical setting, she could have lost touch with her personal values, with the potential of alienation from herself. Her developing self-awareness correlates with the work by Maslow on self-actualisation (Boeree, 2006). Similarly, Knowles (1980), in his work on the dimensions of maturation, discusses an individual's move from superficial to deep concerns, moving away from a focus on particulars towards a focus on principles and from impulsiveness to rationality. This parallels Maslow's idea of differentiating between good and bad from a professional perspective and being unprepared to compromise personal and professional integrity. Olga's ability to deal with problems and challenges illustrates her ability to objectify situations and think more broadly, accepting ambiguity and making choices to invest in dialogue she perceived to be important. Olga was illustrating that she had become more autonomous in her decision-making and enlightened in her view of the world – in other words, she seemed to have integrated her self-identity as a developing health care professional and was more self-accepting of her abilities, strengths and weaknesses. The risk for someone starting out in a health care profession is great; Helkama et al. (2003) discuss a decline and changes in moral reasoning during the education of medical students, while Greenwood (1993), Allcock and Standen (2001) and MacIntosh (2003) discuss possible desensitisation that student nurses undergo during their education, which could have strong moral implications for the quality of care delivered.

In the case of the Dutch participants in Esterhuizen's 2007 research, those who completed the programme, whilst adapting initially to ward cultures, were acutely aware of the fact that they were adapting to something they didn't necessary concur with – they seemed almost to have a strategic approach to their development deciding at which points they were prepared to extend and/or set boundaries. Several authors have referred to this adaptive behaviour, often in the context of reflective practice. Johns and Freshwater (1998), for example, note that many students become disillusioned as the gap between espoused theories and theories in action become more apparent. Achieving the balance between the adaptation of the self (beliefs and values) and the liberation of the self through clinical practice and education is perhaps a constant struggle, but is also an extremely fertile space for growth and transformation.

So far in the discussion, self-awareness has been linked directly to the patient–client relationship. However, cultural knowledge and cues are taken from social context, and learning can occur only through an interaction of the individual with the environment (Knowles, 1980; Kolb, 1984; MacIntosh, 2003). We have already mentioned, albeit tangentially, intuition and knowing, this in the context of presence. The idea of 'just knowing' also resonates with work by Neville (2005) and Leners (1992), in which they discuss elements of intuition. But there was more behind integrating theory and practice than intuition, although it did seem to stand the students in good stead when dealing with issues of power on the wards. One student mentioned that the registered staff 'just radiate' authority, but this could have been her perception of 'authority' versus 'power' and the ultimate reason that she left the programme.

A possible link between a 'negative' occupational socialisation and attrition rates among nurses is easily made. It would seem logical to assume that an 'unsuccessful' socialisation could result in attrition. This cannot be assumed automatically as both Glossop (2002) and Last and Fulbrook (2003) provide various reasons underlying the attrition rate which would probably indicate that a combination of factors are responsible. However, Glossop (2002) suggests from her findings that 17% of students withdrew from the course due to a 'wrong career choice' and 22% provided little or no information as to their reasons for leaving. She also suggests that 56% of the students withdrew during the first 18 months of the course. Last and Fulbrook (2003) establish from their Delphi Study that a 94% majority of the students taking part in the study felt that the programme needed more guidance and structure in the initial phase. The findings of Glossop (2002) and Last and Fulbrook (2003) could then indicate that the experiences of nursing students in their first contact with the educational programme and clinical placement areas raise substantial doubt as to cause them to withdraw from the course. The idea of clinical placements being responsible for the undermining of the nursing students' motivation is contrary to the idea of the workplace being a powerful learning environment, as discussed by Spouse (2001), or a place to learn to care.

■ Should I stay or should I go now?

What, then, is contained in the professional curriculum and initial contact with the practice setting that is causing this attrition rate? Spouse (2000) and Last and Fulbrook (2003) discuss the lack of morale and high degrees of stress among registered nurses in the clinical setting and indicate that students strongly doubted whether they would want to be part of 'such a workforce' in which they would not be able to provide the care they wanted to provide from an ideological point of view. These authors also discuss the students' lack of confidence to practice nursing and link their self-confidence level to the so-called 'theory–practice gap'. Randle (2003) also addresses the issue of the lack of self-confidence and self-esteem, but links this to findings regarding bullying in the clinical setting. Farrell (2001) discusses hierarchical power and the issue of horizontal violence. Both Randle (2003) and Farrell (2001) suggest that victims of bullying or horizontal violence do not speak about their experiences, but prefer to remain anonymous (Freshwater, 2000). This could tie in with the findings published by Glossop (2002), which showed that a large percentage of students left the nursing programme due to its being 'a wrong career choice' or without providing additional information.

The question may rightly be asked as to why nurses then stay in the profession if the clinical experience is so negative. Many of the authors quoted have focused on the negative influences in their studies rather than on what inspires nurses to remain in practice. However, a number of authors refer to interpersonal and interactive relationships as providing the nurse with a positive and inspirational experience (Widdershoven, 1999; Spouse, 2001; Stickley & Freshwater, 2002). Philpin (1999) discusses the influence on student experience in terms of distance from the medical model and indicates the positive experience of nurses working in 'chronic areas' rather than 'acute areas' – students appear to be provided with opportunities for inter-acting with patients and are treated as team members, rather than being subservient. This effect of interacting with the chronically ill appears to place 'care' as a core element of working and learning. This is substanti-ated by Spouse (2000), who describes a situation of attrition with a student returning, at a later date, to a course in which nursing was presented as an art and a science, rather than from a task-oriented or biomedical approach. However, Randle (2002), within the concept of moral identity and practice, discusses the desensitisation of students to ethical and moral issues within the clinical setting.

It would appear that students and nurses adapt or learn to deal with the moral culture of the clinical setting as they progress through their education and careers. The importance of supporting the original ideals of students and registered staff throughout the process of learning and 'becoming professional' is discussed in terms of revisiting and reworking issues over a period of time (Watson et al., 1999; MacIntosh, 2003) – a plea for reflection, reflexivity and a reflective way of being. One way of attempt-ing to sustain moral sensitivity is to provide ongoing reflective workshops as part of the curriculum. During these workshops students are encour-aged and assisted to analyse moral dilemmas relevant to their seniority and appropriate to their experience (Esterhuizen & Kooman, 2001). This approach provides students with a specific focus on their reflection and enhances their self-awareness of fundamental norms and values related to both nursing and their way of being.

■ Coping or mal-adaptation?

The disillusion and trauma of feeling the need to leave nursing can be dev-astating for staff who have reached the point of burnout, and the findings by Tinsley and France (2004) relate the exodus of staff to organisational and peer bullying.

As practitioners, educators and managers in health and social care, we need to ask ourselves whether coping with situations that arise means that we have socialised into a system: in other words, whether socialisation means that we have coped successfully, or whether coping is a temporary method of surviving, a way of 'conning' the environment into believing you've adapted or socialised, only to re-embrace your initial ideas and beliefs once you have the 'freedom' to set your own course. If the latter is true, it implies a system of power and (perceived) oppression. One might argue that learning to cope is part of the socialisation, and indeed edu-cational, process; something we all have to learn in order to survive. As such it is questionable as to whether the process of socialisation can actu-ally be separated from the individual's educational process. Bruner's work discusses the sociological–educational interaction in great detail (Bruner, 1996). He suggests that 'education is not an island, but part of the continent of culture' (Bruner, 1996, p. 11). The interface between the two is clear: education has a role in the culture and the lives of those living in the culture. And, conversely, education 'reflects the distribution of power, status and other benefits'. Bruner argues that culture defines what is thought to be good and of value, and because individuals are part of that culture, they adapt to the demands placed on them by their environment.

■ Conclusion

The way many health and care professionals, now in management and educational roles, have been socialised has a direct impact on the new generation of social professionals that they lead and educate. Sometimes this perpetuates the cycle of oppressive socialisation that is described in the literature. Who is responsible for breaking this cycle? One might argue that this is partly the domain of education. This begs the question: to what extent, within the restraints of our own psyche, do we as educationalists, and indeed the curriculum, allow the natural talents of the individual student or colleague to emerge and support and nurture them to a point of independence in their professional role? If we are able to support and nurture the individual in their development, then the process, rather than the product, must be the focus. This must have an impact on the quality of patient care in which the nurse meets the patient on their own terms, conditions and level (Nåden & Eriksson, 2002; Turkel, 2003; Freshwater & Stickley, 2004). We all have the potential to create a dependant relationship with students and/or colleagues whilst deceiving them into thinking that they are independent and assertive. Neville (2005) and Espeland and Shanta (2001) discuss issues of dependency and counter-transference between lecturer/mentor and student. This is, potentially, a huge risk for both parties and provides yet another slant to the Levinas' discussion concerning self-awareness and 'love' – for want of a better word – for the other. The unconditional positive regard of manager/educator for the practitioner is as important as the practitioner's regard for the patient and provides a strong role model and context for experiential learning. But the idea of learning from reflection goes further. Bruner (1996, p. 19) suggests that

> 'thinking about thinking' has to be a principal ingredient of any empowering practice of education.

The intimacy and vulnerability shared by both parties could be misinterpreted in the closeness of the moment and misconstrued by those outside the relationship, observing from a distance. However, this does not mean that distance and coldness is called for; rather we would argue that the process of reflection and learning from each other through relationship, in terms of both process and content, provides an opportunity to embody, experience and express human agape, that is love.

References

Allcock, N. & Standen, P. 2001. Student nurses' experiences of caring for patients in pain. *International Journal of Nursing Studies*, 38: 287–295.

Arman, M. & Rehnsfeldt, A. 2006. The presence of love in ethical caring. *Nursing Forum*, 41 (1): 4–12.

Becker Hentz, P. & Lauterbach, S. S. 2005. Becoming self-reflective: Caring for self and others. *International Journal for Human Caring*, 9 (1): 24–28.

Bennett, S., Robertson, R. & Moss, P. 1992. Education: Learning the pitfalls of codependency. *Nursing Management*, 25 (2): 80B–80H.

Boeree, C. G. 2006. Personality theories: Abraham Maslow. *Psychology Department: Shippensberg University.* http://www.social-psychology.de/do/pt_maslow.pdf (11 January 2007).

Boykin, A. & Schoenhofer, S. O. 2001. *Nursing as Caring: A Model for Transforming Practice.* Boston: National League for Nursing.

Bruner, J. 1996. *The Culture of Education.* London: Harvard University Press.

Callister, L. C. & Freeborn, D. 2007. Nurse midwives with women: Ways of knowing in nurse midwives. *International Journal for Human Caring*, 11 (1): 8–415.

Chappelle, L. S. & Sorrentino, E. A. 1993. Assessing the co-dependency issues within a nursing environment. *Nursing Management*, 24 (5): 40–44.

Dolan, J. A., Fitzpatrick, M. L. & Herrmann, E. K. 1983. *Nursing in Society. A Historical Perspective.* Philadelphia: W.B. Saunders Co.

Driscoll, J. 2000. *Practising Clinical Supervision.* London: Baillière Tindall.

Ekebergh, M., Lepp, M. & Dahlberg, K. 2004. Reflective learning with drama in nursing education – A Swedish attempt to overcome the theory praxis gap. *Nurse Education Today*, 24 (8): 622–628.

Elliott, M. 2002. The clinical environment: A source of stress for undergraduate nurses. *Australian Journal of Advanced Nursing*, 20 (1): 34–38.

Espeland, K. & Shanta, L. 2001. Empowering versus enabling in academia. *Journal of Nursing Education*, 40 (8): 342–346.

Esterhuizen, P. & Kooyman, A. 2001. Empowering moral decision making in nurses. *Nurse Education Today*, 21: 640–647.

Esterhuizen, P. 1996. Is the professional code still the cornerstone of professional practice? *Journal of Advanced Nursing*, 53 (1): 104–110.

Esterhuizen, P. 2007. *The Journey from Neophyte to Registered Nurse – A Dutch Experience.* Unpublished doctoral thesis. Bournemouth: University of Bournemouth.

Farrell, G. A. 2001. From tall poppies to squashed seeds: Why don't nurses pull together more? *Journal of Advanced Nursing*, 35 (1): 26–33.

Finch, L. P. 2006. Patients' communication with nurses: Relational communication and preferred nurse behaviours. *International Journal for Human Caring*, 10 (4): 14–22.

Freshwater, D. 1998. *Transformatory Learning in Nurse Education.* PhD thesis. Nottingham: University of Nottingham.

Freshwater, D. 2000. Crosscurrents: against cultural narration in nursing. *Journal of Advance Nursing*, 32 (2), 481–484.

Freshwater, D. 2002. *Therapeutic Nursing: Improving Patient Care through Self Awareness and Reflection.* London: Sage.

Freshwater, D. & Robertson, C. 2002. *Emotion and Need.* Open University Press, Milton Keynes.

Freshwater, D. & Stickley, T. 2004. The heart of the art: Emotional intelligence in nurse education. *Nursing Inquiry*, 11 (2): 91–98.

Gilmartin, J. 2000. Psychodynamic sources of resistance among student nurses: some observation in a human relations context. *Journal of Advanced Nursing*, 32 (6), 1533–1541.

Glossop, C. 2002. Student nurse attrition: Use of an exit-interview procedure to determine students' leaving reasons. *Nurse Education Today*, 22: 375–386.

Greenwood, J. 1993. The apparent desensitization of student nurses during their professional socialization: A cognitive perspective. *Journal of Advanced Nursing*, 18: 1471–1479.

Helkama, K., Uutela, A., Pohjanheimo, E., Salminen, S., Kaponen, A. & Rantanen-Väntsi, L. 2003. Moral reasoning and values in medical school: A longitudinal study in Finland. *Scandinavian Journal of Educational Research*, 47 (4): 399–411.

Hopkins, L. M. & Jackson, W. 2002. Revisiting the issue of co-dependency in nursing: Caring or caretaking? *Canadian Journal of Nursing*, 34 (4): 35–46.

Johns, C. 1998. Caring through a reflective lens: Giving meaning to being a reflective practitioner. *Nursing Inquiry*, 5: 18–24.

Johns, C. 2001. Depending on the intent and emphasis of the supervisor, clinical supervision can be a different experience. *Journal of Nursing Management*, 9, 139–145.

Johns, C. 2002. *Guided Reflection: Advancing Practice*. Oxford: Blackwell Science Ltd.

Knowles, M. S. 1980. *The Modern Practice of Adult Education: From Pedagogy to Andragogy*. New Jersey: Prentice-Hall, Engelwood-Cliffs.

Kolb, D. 1984. *Experiential Learning*. New Jersey: Prentice-Hall, Engelwood-Cliffs.

Last, L. & Fulbrook, P. 2003. Why do student nurses leave? Suggestions from a Delphi Study. *Nurse Education Today*, 23: 449–458.

Leners, D. W. 1992. Intuition in nursing practice: Deep connections. *Journal of Holistic Nursing*, 6 (10): 137–153.

Levinas, E. 1991. *Entre Nous* (translated by M. B. Smith & B. Harshav). London: Continuum.

Leyshon, S. 2002. Empowering practitioners: An unrealistic expectation of nurse education? *Journal of Advanced Nursing*, 40 (4): 466–474.

Maben, J., Latter, S. and Macleod Clark, J. 2007. The sustainability of ideals, values and the nursing mandate: Evidence from a longitudinal qualitative study. *Nursing Inquiry*, 14 (2): 99–113.

MacIntosh, J. 2003. Reworking professional nursing identity. *Western Journal of Nursing Research*, 25 (6): 725–741.

Malloy, G. B. & Berkery, A. C. 1993. Co-dependency: A feminist perspective. *Journal of Psychosocial Nursing*, 31 (4), 15–19.

Martsolf, D. S. 2002. Codependency, boundaries, and professional nurse caring. *Orthopaedic Nursing*, 21 (6), 61–67.

Mc Cabe, C. & Timmins, F. 2003. Teaching assertiveness to undergraduate nursing students. *Nurse Education in Practice*, 3 (1): 30–42.

Nåden, D. 2002. Confirmation and encounter – Two fundamental categories in nursing as an art: Perceptions and reflections on caring. *Keynote address: 7th International Reflective Practice Conference: Reflecting on Reflective Practice*. June 6th–8th, 2002. Egmond aan Zee, Netharlands.

Nåden, D. & Eriksson, K. 2000. The phenomenon of confirmation: An aspect of nursing as an art. *International Journal for Human Caring*, 4 (3): 23–28.

Nåden, D. & Eriksson, K. 2002. Encounter: A fundamental category of nursing as an art. *International Journal for Human Caring*, 6 (1): 34–40.

Nåden, D. & Eriksson, K. 2004. Understanding the importance of values and moral attitudes in nursing care in preserving human dignity. *Nursing Science Quarterly*, 17 (1): 86–91.

Neville, B. 2005. *Educating Psyche: Emotion, Imagination and the Unconscious in Learning.* Greensborough (Aus.): Flat Chat Press.

Philpin, S. M. 1999. The impact of 'Project 2000' educational reforms on occupational socialization of nurses: An exploratory study. *Journal of Advanced Nursing,* 29 (6): 1326–1331.

Randle, J. 2002. The shaping of moral identity and practice. *Nurse Education in Practice,* 2: 251–256.

Randle, J. 2003. Bullying in the nursing profession. *Journal of Advanced Nursing,* 43 (4): 395–401.

Shearer, R. & Davidhizar, R. 2003. Educational innovations: Using role play to develop cultural competence. *Journal of Nursing Education,* 42 (6): 273–276.

Simons, L., Herbert, L., Tee, S., Lathlean, J., Burgess, A. & Gibson, C. 2006. Integrated service user-led teaching in higher education: Experiences and learning points. *Mental Health Review,* 11: 14–18.

Smith, P. & Gray, B. 2001. Emotional labour of nursing revisited: Caring and learning 2000. *Nurse Education in Practice,* 1: 42–49.

Spence, D. J. 2001. Prejudice, paradox, and possibility: Nursing people from cultures other than our own. *Journal of Transcultural Nursing,* 12 (2): 100–106.

Spouse, J. 2000. An impossible dream? Images of nursing held by pre-registration students and their effect on sustaining motivation to become nurses. *Journal of Advanced Nursing,* 32 (3): 730–739.

Spouse, J. 2001. Workplace learning: Pre-registration nursing students' perspectives. *Nurse Education in Practice,* 1: 149–156.

Stickley, T. & Freshwater, D. 2002. The art of loving and the therapeutic relationship. *Nursing Inquiry,* 9 (4): 250–256.

Tanyi, R. A. 2002. Towards clarification of the meaning of spirituality. *Journal of Advanced Nursing,* 39 (5): 500–509.

Taylor, B. 1994. *Being Human: Ordinariness in Nursing.* Melbourne: Churchill Livingstone.

Tinsley, C. & France, N. E. M. 2004. The trajectory of the registered nurse's exodus from the profession: A phenomenological study of the lived experience of oppression. *International Journal for Human Caring,* 8 (1), 8–12.

Turkel, M. 2003. A journey onto caring as experienced by nurse managers. *International Journal for Human Caring,* 7 (1): 20–26.

von Dietze, E. & Orb, A. 2000. Compassionate care: A moral dimension of nursing. *Nursing Inquiry,* 7 (3): 166–174.

Warne, T. & McAndrew, S. 2004. *Nursing, Nurse Education and Professionalisation in a Contemporary Context.* In: T. Warne & S. McAndrew (eds.) *Using Patient Experience in Nurse Education.* Hampshire: Palgrave MacMillan.

Watson, J. 1988. *Nursing: Human Science and Human Care. A Theory of Nursing.* New York: National League for Nursing.

Watson, J. 1998. A meta-reflection on reflective practice and caring theory. In: C. Johns & D. Freshwater (eds.) *Transforming Nursing through Reflective Practice.* 214–220. Oxford: Blackwell Science.

Watson, R., Deary, I. J. & Lea, A. 1999. A longitudinal study into the perceptions of caring and nursing among student nurses. *Journal of Advanced Nursing,* 29 (5): 1228–1237.

Widdershoven, G. A. M. 1999. Care, cure and interpersonal understanding. *Journal of Advanced Nursing,* 29 (5): 1163–1169.

Yates, J. G. & Mc Daniel, J. L. 1994. Are you losing yourself in co-dependency? *American Journal of Nursing,* April: 32–36.

Chapter 14

Facilitating new worlds? Deaf people's access to nurse education

Naomi Sharples

■ Introduction

It is well documented in sociological literature that any threat to an existing social order is likely to cause fear, misunderstanding and anxiety. The consequence for those who threaten the existing order could be isolation and/or marginalisation (Clarke, 1999). A person who by the nature of their difference undermines the prevailing social order will become the target of persecution with their difference being used to legitimise acts of exclusion (Clarke, 1999; Bauman, 1990). The unacceptability of being different can often result in social exclusion and 'outsiderness' (Smith, 1992). Outsiderness can be experienced because of differences – for example, physical, sexual, cultural, or racial – which set an individual apart from the prevailing social discourse. This chapter draws upon an exploration of the way in which the Deaf Peoples Access to Nurse Education (DPANE) project provided opportunity for one group of 'excluded' people to gain access to education, leading to qualification for professional practice. Whilst this chapter focuses on deaf people becoming qualified nurses, the principles discussed in this chapter can be applied to other health and social care contexts where individuals experience a sense of difference and outsiderness.

Deaf people form a community of approximately 50,000 people in Britain; this community is made up of a shared language, experiences, education, humour and history. The community is not homogenous, nor is it easily understood. It is made up of deaf people from deaf families, deaf people from hearing families and hearing people with strong connections to deaf people through family ties or by their work within the deaf community. There are those who would contest that hearing people could ever be full members of the deaf community because of their audiological status whilst others have a more inclusive view of 'community'. Despite the contested membership of this small community it is very clear that deaf people have experienced degrees of empowerment and disempowerment throughout history with hearing people as the protagonists in this narrative. Such narratives are exemplified in terms of deaf people's involvement as providers and recipients of health and social care services.

The chapter explores both the educational world of deaf people and the concept of education as a tool for empowerment, and explores the link between education and communication and their relationship to emancipation. Utilising these explorations, the chapter provides an overview of the practical issues facing tutors and mentors who work with Deaf students in education and practice settings.

■ Background

Throughout this chapter the nurses will be referred to as deaf nurses or nurses who use sign language as their first or preferred language. This chapter is drawn from my experience of leading the DPANE project, which ran from 2000 to 2006. This project was initiated by lead nurses from the National Mental Health Services for Deaf People in Manchester, Birmingham and London. In each of these services deaf people were employed alongside hearing people to support people within the British deaf population who required specific mental health services. Each of the above services has an in-patient and community service, and the majority of the deaf people employed in the services worked in assistant or support roles. A minority of the deaf employees worked in professional role such as psychologist, social workers or teachers. At the conception of the project there were no qualified deaf nurses working in the services because support systems for student nurses who were deaf did not exist in higher education institutions; the necessary financial resources were inaccessible to people whose first language is sign language and who would require interpreters and note takers to access nurse education as it is currently provided.

Thus deaf people continued to work as Health Care Assistants (HCAs) despite some having the capacity and capability to access higher education. Due to the 'glass ceiling' effect the services lost valuable and experienced HCAs to other areas of employment where a lack of a professional qualification did not preclude people from lead positions within their organisations. Such inequity served as a motivation for health professionals in delivering deaf-centred services where the language of the services is sign language and where deaf culture is understood and celebrated.

■ In with the out group

During the 1960s and 1970s, mental health services specifically for deaf people were being established in Europe and America. The momentum for service development came from people such as Dr John Denmark. As a child John Denmark had grown up with the pupils in his fathers' school for deaf children, learning about deaf people and also learning sign language. On becoming a psychiatrist he began to identify a number of deaf people isolated on wards, without access to communication, lost and alienated within an already alien environment. In order to meet the needs of these individuals he established the first mental health service for deaf people (Denmark, 1994). This raises the question of what makes a person want to work within another culture/community, which is a complicated issue. We are often made to feel alien as visitors to other groups, a position that is uncomfortable and yet for some people there is a strong urge to make a difference. There are complicated reasons for out-group behaviour such as this, and Borshuk (2004) suggests that educational attainment, being from middle or upper class and being privileged, may help the out-group person to identify inequity in society and also provide the means and motivation to act in order to effect the current inequitable situation. This position is interesting when one considers that for deaf people educational attainment can be so illusive and dependent on external influences so much more than for hearing people no matter what their class.

■ A brief journey through the history of deaf education and employment

To understand where we are now we must understand what has gone before, and what influences our current education and health perspectives. A starting point is the exploration of the social and religious concepts of 'voice'. As individuals, members of society, we acknowledge the sense or belief that having no voice is essentially disempowering. On one level it is clear that without a voice an individual is rendered weakened and unable to participate within wider society. We are inundated by the idea that we should be giving people, groups and communities their 'voice' through consultation and by 'putting the individual at the centre' of the issue and 'listening' to them. However, there needs to be a shared language and shared access to information that would promote the individual's decision-making process and enable the individual to express themselves. Without being enabled one becomes 'disabled' from society by those who have a voice and thus the knowledge and power.

It is clear that when faced with such a 'disabled' minority individuals within the majority become motivated to seek solutions that are focused on changing the individual, making the individual 'fit', or providing robust arguments in support of disbarring the individual from aspects of life that would require a voice. The manner in which this is achieved can be disguised as 'care' or 'control' depending on the zeitgeist of the time.

Whilst agreement prevails that to be empowered one requires a 'voice', where that voice is denied the individual is unable to participate in the debate. Fundamentally, they do not partake in the development of understanding in the world through the generation of symbolic representation of thoughts, ideas and concepts. In a world of sign language deaf people do have a voice and non-signers are at a disadvantage, a worthy learning experience for anyone new to deaf culture. Today, a minimum of 50,000 deaf people in Britain use British Sign Language (BSL) as their first or preferred language. BSL was recognised as an official British language in March 2003.

■ Learning to get a voice

When reflecting on deaf history there are times where there have been significant paradigm shifts. In the 18th and 19th centuries there were teachers of deaf children who were themselves deaf, so providing empowering influences for the deaf community. During this period the debate between the oralists and the supporters of sign language continued. This debate was cut short in Milan in 1888. The 'Milan Conference' is seen as a turning point in deaf education and it is a watershed that still provokes intense reactions in deaf people today. The conference challenged educators to look at the success of students trained in oral methods, and faced with a group of deaf students who could speak and understand speech in a number of languages, education took a significant turn towards oralism. Sign language was not supported because of the lack of acceptance that sign languages were true languages. However, with many paradigm shifts the majority get anxious and change can be toppled by the might of societies' need to find equilibrium. Thomas Kuhn suggested that the anxiety produced by new understandings can send the old-order thinkers to develop protectionist behaviours meted against new-order thinkers (Bird, 2005).

Linguistically, we know that sign language has the same functions and capabilities as oral languages; scientifically, the debate could support sign language. Socially, the paradigm shifts according to the *Weltanschauung* of the day. On both sides of the debate hostility is high; for the educationalists, medics and geneticists there is also the support to be gained from powerful positions within society, not so for the deaf individuals, who, in the maelstrom, lose their 'voice' by losing their language. Jurgen Habermas identifies the concept of 'communicative power' suggesting that society's institutions should be the channel for the voice of individuals within society, this channel funnelling individuals' opinions to thus inform and change society. For deaf people, their channels have been stifled and unfulfilling due to the communities' lack of such communicative power.

It was the bureaucratisation of deaf education policies and laws in the twentieth century which brought about change rather than the strength of individuals or groups of people determined to empower deaf people (Branson and Miller, 2002). Education allows and encourages individuals to understand their society and function within it through the empowerment provided by knowledge. This position is one pursued by Brazilian educationalist Paulo Freire and has its origins within the philosophy of Hegel and Marx. However, this emancipatory approach had little hold on British education and even less in the education of deaf children. It is this emancipatory position that most resonates with the deaf people's access to nurse education project because despite the movement against sign language, and as a credit to the deaf community, change was slowly underway.

With the continued development of establishments within the deaf community such as churches, schools, colleges and deaf clubs more deaf people began to gravitate towards these centres and sign language began to thrive within the deaf milieu. With language came culture, humour, poetry, art, drama, history and a strong sense of in-group and out-group politics. Such language development of oppressed people is, as Barthes (1993) suggests, a 'transitive language of emancipation', a way of describing the community and the environment in which it exists. A political movement was developing within the deaf community, the movement basing its identity on being a linguistic minority group rather than on the concept of disability (Padden and Humphries, 1988).

The 1960s and 1970s witnessed the development of bilingualism as a preferred method of education supported by the recognition of sign languages as true languages and the failure of oralism for some children. Deaf children were not attaining on a par with hearing children. The average deaf school-leaver had a reading age of eight years. However, deaf children of deaf parents were managing to achieve qualifications, and research into other bilingual communities was suggesting great opportunity for deaf children (Gregory, 1996). In the 1980s and 1990s there were wide variations in the educational approaches for children. The emphasis is now on mainstreaming deaf children with peripatetic or specific classroom support. There are some specific schools that educate deaf children which tend to focus on children who are particularly bright or those who have more complex needs.

■ Education as a tool for empowerment

Deaf people, particularly women, had often poor experiences of education (Walsh, 1996). The curriculum was often designed to enable the young adult to 'survive' in society rather than enabling the young person to access learning through visual language. Interestingly, the Galludet University in Washington, a university established for deaf students, saw their first deaf president in 1988 following years of hearing people holding the power position. The revolution gave rise to concepts such as 'Deaf Power' that spurred change on the other side of the Atlantic. Moves towards empowerment were supported by the work of linguists Edward Klima and Ursula Bellugi (1979). Deaf people had a sense of being recognised; their language was accepted as a true language not a gestured version of spoken English despite opposition from people as influential as Noam Chomsky (Sacks, 1989). Universities in Britain began to develop Deaf Studies Departments; the first was established in Bristol with the Universities of Central Lancashire and Wolverhampton following closely behind. Sign language classes spread throughout further education colleges becoming the second most popular night class; only information technology classes fared better.

The work of Paulo Freire encapsulates the emancipation of oppressed people through education. Significantly, Freire states that understanding the reasons for oppression is in itself not enough; one has to act on this understanding to change the situation. Working as an educator in Brazil in the 1950s and 1960s and again in the 1980s, Freire focused his work on bringing literacy to the masses of workers who had never experienced literacy before. Firstly, his literacy campaign was established in order for workers to be able to participate in the political elections; to vote you had to be literate. In the 1980s Freire went on to establish a literacy programme in Brazil which created a vision of democratic education that challenged the didactic 'empty vessel' approach to learning. Such emancipation requires knowledge gained through dialogue and a 'communicative act' which is reflective of the history of the students' world and the 'gnosiological' or real-world understanding (Gadotti, 2007). Citizenship, and multicultural democracy through inclusion, was a foundation stone for Freire and is mirrored in the DPANE project, which incorporates social, medical, linguistic and cultural parameters.

■ DPANE

For some, the DPANE project pioneered the empowerment of the deaf community and at the same time facilitated access to the educational playing field for deaf people through technology and human aids to communication (such as interpreters and note takers). Nyatanga and Dann (2002) propose that empowerment is a process and an outcome that involves people drawing power from inside themselves in order to have a voice and that this voice provides influence and power over important aspects of their lives. Importantly, Nyatanga and Dann (2002) clearly express that one cannot empower another; one can only transform factors within the environment that will facilitate the individual or group to develop the strength from within to change their circumstances.

Jurgen Habermas argues that to be emancipated individuals need to be free and able to express themselves, to communicate with each other in order to interact with each other and their environment. This freedom of communication and social interaction enables individuals to understand and change their current situation making use of advances in science and technology.

This view of emancipation resonates deeply within the DPANE project. It is a motivator and acts as an idealised framework in which to establish good practice. However, empowering deaf people by enabling access to health and social care education could be seen as merely emancipating an individual from one position only for them to become disempowered in their next position. As such it could be argued that education only ever offers choice; it does not offer emancipation because the society that has created the environment able to sustain the inclusion of a once excluded community also manages and monitors the educational, health, welfare and legal contexts where levels of individual empowerment are questionable.

The ultimate aim of the project was to benefit deaf clients within mental health services by providing qualified key workers who shared their linguistic and cultural background. These key workers in turn would move into more senior positions within the organisation, which would facilitate greater understanding of deaf people's needs at an organisational level.

The project was established within the School of Nursing at the University of Salford and the aim was to create an accessible learning environment for deaf people within nurse education. Central to the project being successful was the importance of identifying any barriers that may exist for students accessing the clinical and educational environments. Where there were barriers the project lead needed to develop innovative solutions to establish new ways of working. Peter Senge's concept of a learning organisation provides a framework from which to reflect and articulate the process. Within his framework Senge identifies personal mastery, mental models, team learning and building a shared vision as integral artefacts in the process of organisational learning.

☐ Personal mastery

Personal mastery involves developing the mental and spiritual process that is necessary for a life of continual learning, where one knows one will never arrive at the place of having learnt enough. Reflection and reflective practice is a vital component of personal mastery, as is the ability to use meta-cognitive skills, learning about learning and learning how to learn effectively and efficiently in order to pursue change and progress into new areas of being.

Reflecting on the project, the people involved and the students who are now qualified and in leadership positions has offered a multitude of new perspectives; the one that stands out most clearly is simple. What one individual student needs, and how they will access their clinical or teaching environment, will always be different from the next. What works for one student will not necessarily work for another. This should not be surprising when we just consider the different family expectations, linguistic competencies, communication skills and access to education experiences students have had before they arrive on a health or social care programme. In our risk-focused world it was assumed that we had developed a risk assessment to ensure students were 'safe' to go into clinical practice. Firstly, we have never 'risk-assessed' a student; it is impossible as a hearing person to assess a deaf person's ability (or rather inability as risk assessments tend to look for the negative) to access their environment. Secondly, we have never risk-assessed hearing students who go into deaf clinical environments and this has never created a problem. We do work with clinical placements to support the students in practice and we do have a dedicated tutor who will spend time with clinical teams to discuss access issues.

☐ Mental models

Mental models are our deeply held beliefs and understanding of the world; in this case people's deeply held beliefs and assumptions of 'nurse'. Changing a mental model required current assumptions to be examined and explored with others in relation to their effectiveness or ineffectiveness as a mental model for contemporary nursing. Challenging the stereotypical views of nurses was managed on a number of levels. Firstly, through the provision of information-giving sessions, where the history of deaf people's experiences of hearing hospitals and their crucial role within deaf environments was discussed. Secondly, through conversation with colleagues who were confident to ask questions and start to challenge their own mental models to begin to include signing people within those models and to begin to consider a 'visual' voice. Finally we also needed to establish influences within the systems that support a student's journey through the programme. Systems for recruitment, admission, assessment and clinical placement allocation all needed to take note of and action new ways of working to meet the access needs of deaf student nurses.

☐ Team learning

The dialogue that develops from new and emerging issues forms the basis of team learning. Where team learning occurs change in behaviours filter through the organisation; for example, learning how different it is to work in a classroom where a visual and auditory language requires the supportive platform of using an interpreter. However, this is not always easy; for example, one member of the nursing team thought it would be a better idea for the deaf students, the note taker and the interpreter to sit at the back of the classroom because the signing was 'putting the hearing students off'. By gently asking practical questions such as 'do you think it might be difficult for the interpreter to hear from the back of the lecture hall?' or 'what message do you think that would send to all the students?' or 'what evidence do you have to suggest the hearing students are being put off?' often prompts people to reconsider their practical, well-intentioned solutions. Team learning takes a great deal of time and reinforcement because students move on, staff change and new staff come, and because deaf students do not attend constantly, people forget good practice and inclusive arrangements may fall by the wayside. Individuals need to know who is responsible for what aspect of the deaf students' needs.

☐ Building a shared vision

Strangely building a shared vision is often easier outside your organisation than within it. For example, people who attend a national conference focused on disability and access to education are more likely to understand the project than a colleague in the same school as the project. Within the school, the building of a shared vision has been successful, whereby professional body reviews and institutional reviews have all supported and promoted the project. At an individual level there have been greater challenges in building the shared vision of an accessible supportive learning environment for deaf people. Some of these challenges include the number of students and staff, time and expertise.

The number of students is critical when gaining a sense of change, difference and shared image. Where there are groups of deaf students in a cohort their experience is much improved. Single students are often well supported by their peers but can become invisible to organisational mechanisms.

The number of staff involved with the students is also a critical factor: too few and the responsibility for the students always lies at their door, they become the 'deaf tutors'; too many and the critical mass is compromised, people can abdicate responsibility, leaving the students unsupported and without access. Of course this is a situation likely to be found in many other educational contexts.

Time is particularly pertinent when learning to work in new ways. For example, the amount of time it takes to engage with individual tutors and support staff in order to develop their knowledge and skills of working with those who are deaf is greater than the time needed to present information and ideas to others at a national conference.

Expertise often equates to the technical aspects of building a relationship with others; for example, the acquisition and use of a language to communicate. However, this can result in the 'deaf tutor' outcome noted above. Expertise that is represented in the tutor's ability to effectively engage with the students' perspective is crucial. Technical expertise can lead to a position where students are seen to fit in with everyone else; that their being in the school has become the norm and everything is fine now and the need to recognise their difference is lost. The numbers, time and expertise equation relates directly to the concept of voice and community.

When there is a clear presence, where time is allocated and used effectively and where expertise is valued, the students have a voice, they have improved access to the programme, their learning experience is enhanced and their skills and knowledge developed.

☐   The process

Four students were recruited to start the course in September 2000, with another three recruited in 2002, two students in 2003 and two students in 2004. A nurse lecturer with knowledge of the project, the deaf community and sign language skills was recruited to provide support for the students, University staff and placement supervisors and their teams. This person was the main point of contact for providing support on deaf awareness, cultures, communities, languages and services, so that the needs of the students are met. A project administrator, sign language interpreters and note takers have also been recruited to support the students. Students also make use of IT equipment, study skills tutorials and clinical tutorials, most of which are now paid for through the Disabled Students' Allowance. Practice placements are mostly within deaf services, acute provision, community, child and adolescent mental health, and forensic services, including high-secure provision placements. Some students also access hearing services to support their learning. Where this occurs the student has an interpreter with them as much as they need.

The students who are deaf learn with hearing colleagues in mixed groups. The diversity within the groups offers great learning opportunities for all students. Students are encouraged to adhere to skilled communication practices to ensure that the classroom communication is accessible for students and interpreters. These practices include clear turn-taking in discussions, avoiding speaking or signing over each other to ensure everyone is heard. The group facilitator, whether this person is a tutor or student, needs to be visually vigilant to see when someone wants to make a point, to indicate gently who will be speaking or signing next. This is a very active skill demanded by all the students who need to be heard.

Working with interpreters has been both rewarding and challenging for all concerned. The trainee and qualified interpreters who work with the tutors and students are professionals in their own rights and as such are determined to provide full access for the students. This access is enhanced by them working in pairs to avoid becoming tired and ineffective and having access to each session plan, and as much theoretical content is given before the session occurs so that they can read up on the subject area in order to offer a fuller and more rich interpretation. Interpreters are bound by their code of ethics to say something if the communication process is undermining any of the participants. It can be hurtful to lecturers to realise they may not be providing full access; however, if they consider the interpreters the experts in these matters it becomes more of a partnership in the classroom.

Lecturers who can provide explanations and examples of application of theory to practice not only assist the students in the classroom but also support the interpretation process. It must be recognised that any new concept in health and social care demands a new sign in BSL. The students, interpreters and tutors have to be prepared to negotiate their way though the process of developing new signs, new vocabulary, a heavy responsibility but one that will not be taken up by anyone else.

All lecturers involved with the deaf students need to understand practical issues such as how interpreters are booked and how long ahead a booking needs to take place. They need to be aware that if videos are being used they need to be subtitled. If they are not subtitled the interpreters need to see it before the session so they know how to interpret the content. We have found that working with a core of approximately six interpreters who know the programme, the students and the staff, is the most appropriate way to meet our needs.

All sessions are also supported by note takers, who take notes of the lecture, discussions and debate within the classroom for the deaf student to refer to again later. Notes are often used as an aide mémoir for the students to re-visualise a point, or re-engage with a scenario in the classroom. Again the lecturer needs to be aware of the needs of the note takers, pace the session, draw clear points, reiterate information if necessary and be available to provide guidance on meanings. The note takers and the interpreters are necessary additions to the classroom; however, they do not become engaged in the lecture, they are not there to provide opinions, and they do not become involved in discussions unless the discussions are about the communication process. This is in no way meant to disempower the individuals but to allow them to do their complex and demanding roles. Where possible the students choose or make their preferred interpreters known. Where possible the university Equalities Office takes the preferences into account when booking the interpreting service. There is a lead interpreter with whom I can discuss issues, access to material or specific problems. He provides an interpreter perspective and I provide a lecturer perspective and we see where they align or where there may be areas for work.

■ Conclusion

The project has developed over the past eight years and now there are a number of qualified deaf nurses working in the deaf services throughout Britain and providing support for their deaf colleagues. More people from the deaf community are stepping forward to realise their potential to become a health or social care professional. Slowly the deaf community is waking up to the new professionals in their midst.

References

Barthes, R. (1993). *Mythologies*. Vintage Press: London.

Bird, A. (2005). 'Thomas Kuhn', *The Stanford Encyclopaedia of Philosophy* (Spring 2005 Edition), Edward N. Zalta (ed.), ⟨http://plato.stanford.edu/archives/spr2005/entries/thomas-kuhn/⟩.

Bauman, Z. (1990). *Thinking Sociologically*. Oxford: Blackwell.

Borshuk, C. (2004). An interpretive investigation into motivations for out group activism. *The Qualitative Report.* 9(2), June 2004, 300–319. http://www.nova.edu/ssss/QR/QR9-2/borshuk.pdf.

Branson, J. and Miller, D. (2002). *Damned for their Difference. The Cultural Construction of Deaf People as Disabled*. Galludet University Press: USA.

Clarke, S. (1999). Splitting Difference: Psychoanalysis, Hatred and Exclusion. *Journal for the Theory of Social Behaviour*, 29, 121–135.

Denmark, J. C. (1994). *Deafness and Mental Health*. JKP Publications: London.

Gadotti, M. accessed (2007). *Paulo Freire Pedagogy and Democratisation Process in Brazil*. Some aspects of his theory, method and praxis to introduce a debate. www.paulofreire.org/Moacir_Gadotti/Artigos/Ingles/On_Freire/PF_Pedagogy_democratization_in_Brazil_2003.pdf.

Gregory, S. (1996). 'Bilingualism and the Education of Deaf Children: Advances in Practice', a conference held at the University of Leeds June 29th 1996.

Jordan, I. King (2003). Ethical Issues in the Genetic Study of Deafness. *Sign Language Studies*. 4(1, Fall), 4–9, *Gallaudet University Press*.

Klima, E. and Bellugi, U. (1979). *The Signs of Language*. Harvard University Press: USA.

Nyatanga, L. and Dann, K. (2002). Empowerment in nursing: The role of philosophical and psychological factors. *Nursing Philosophy*. 3, 234–239.

Padden, C. and Humphries, T. (1988). *Deaf in America. Voices from a Culture*. Harvard Press: USA.

Sacks, O. (1989). *Seeing Voices: A Journey into the World of the Deaf*. Pan Books: London.

Smith, A. M. (1992). *New right discourses on race and sexuality*. Cambridge University Press: Cambridge.

Walsh, V. (1996). *Breaking Boundaries. Women in Higher Education*. Taylor and Francis: London.

Chapter 15

Lost to transition: Bridging the gap and supporting newly qualified practitioners

Mike Hazelton, Rachel Rossiter and Ellen Sinclair

■ Introduction

> I like coming here actually. I find it therapeutic...but a learning thing as well...It has made me see I did the right thing (new graduate nurse in a group mentorship session).

Recent reports on nurse education and health workforce planning in Australia have pointed to difficulties faced by new graduate nurses in adjusting to the demands of work, and recruitment and retention problems in the nursing workforce. These problems appear to be global, affecting different disciplines and some areas of health and social care more than others. Reducing attrition in the first few years after completing university is an important step towards retaining registered nurses in areas of health and social care that struggles to attract new graduates (Holmes, 2006; Mental Health Nurse Education Taskforce, 2008).

One way of supporting new graduates is through the provision of structured mentorship programmes. The broad purpose of such programmes is to improve care and to enable the health and social care workforce to establish, maintain and promote standards and innovations in practice in the interests of consumers. Whilst this chapter reports on the main findings of a study of group mentorship for new graduate nurses working in one mental health service in New South Wales, Australia, the underlying principles could be applied to differing groups of health and social care professionals.

■ Transition to the workforce

In recent decades a now extensive literature has pointed to the transition from the final year of university study to the first few years in the workforce as a time of conflict and tension for many new graduate nurses (Moorhouse, 1992; Clinton et al., 2001; Commonwealth of Australia, 2002). In addition, numerous reports on nurse education and training and workforce planning have drawn attention to a connection between the difficulties many new graduates experience in adjusting to the demands of work and recruitment and retention problems in the nursing workforce (Clinton et al., 2001; Commonwealth of Australia, 2002; Australian Health Workforce Advisory Committee, 2003). Such changes from student to qualified professional are not confined to nurses, however. For many health and social care professionals, dealing effectively with what Kramer (1974) once referred to as 'reality shock'; working through disillusionment when classroom ideals don't easily match actual work conditions and priorities, can be difficult. Likewise, dealing with the pressure to conform to sometimes questionable work practices and learning to manage time effectively have all been identified as important to the ways in which new graduates develop a secure sense of self as competent professionals (Cobal, 1998). While the nursing shortage has affected all areas of health and social care, both locally and abroad, one service that has been severely affected is that of mental health (Clinton et al., 2001; Mental Health Nurse Education Taskforce, 2008), with perhaps less than 10% of all new graduate nurses expressing an interest in mental health services (Farrell and Carr, 1996). Reducing attrition in the first few years after completing university studies is an important step towards retaining registered nurses in an area of health care that is already undersubscribed by new graduate nurses.

■ The work-readiness of new graduate nurses

Much of the debate surrounding education for health and social care practice turns on concerns over *work-readiness* or the extent to which new graduates are able to 'hit the floor running' when they commence initial employment as qualified professionals (Kilstoff and Rochester, 2003).

For example, and drawing on the findings of the Scoping Study of the Australian Mental Health Nursing Workforce (Clinton and Hazelton 2001a, 2001b, 2001c, 2001d, 2002) it is argued that Australian universities have largely failed to prepare undergraduate students as beginning practitioners of mental health nursing; that the quality of education in mental health nursing in Australian universities was constrained by a lack of clinical placements of sufficient quality and by competition for clinical placements among students of various health professions. Whilst the quality of mental health nursing content and experience is improving in some universities, planning and development of the mental health nursing workforce is seen to be inadequate in ensuring that the future needs of specialist mental health services will be met; and closer collaboration between health and education is required if there is to be any progress in the preparation of the mental health nursing workforce.

Addressing similar concerns, the Australian Universities Teaching Committee (AUTC) report on Outcomes and Curriculum Development in Major Health Care Disciplines (2003) summarised best practice in health–education alliances that optimise clinical learning as including the provision of quality preceptorship for students for each placement; the provision of mentoring and role-modelling by experienced health care professionals; an environment of practical realism that links theory and practice; the consolidation of clinical learning experiences; and continuing the development and use of innovative clinical practicum models that promote teaching and facilitate learning (Clare et al., 2003).

To date, considerable attention has been given to 'fixing' the health care professional problem at the level of undergraduate education. The basic assumption here is that it ought to be possible to redesign training programmes to be more relevant to workforce needs, thus attracting more practically minded young people into the health and social care professions. For example, the issues facing undergraduate nurse education seem to be very similar to those experienced by new graduate nurses, including the provision of quality mentoring and role-modelling by experienced registered nurses; the opportunity to work in clinical environments characterised by practical realism that links theory and practice; and the opportunity to be involved in service development models promoting evidence-based practice and the development of new models of care.

■ Mentorship and clinical supervision

Revisiting such programmes also provide opportunities for consideration of ethical issues (Gabbard, 1997). The approach adopted can be individual- or group-based. Group-based approaches combine the cost-effectiveness of reducing the amount of time in which staff are absent from clinical areas with the benefits of shared reflection on participants' values, knowledge, experiences, thoughts and feelings (Berg and Hallberg, 2000).

Mentoring and clinical supervision are also frequently raised in discussions of how to address problems in the health and social care workforce. Clinical supervision has been reported to assist in the development of professionalism (Lindahl and Norberg, 2002) and the maintenance of professional standards (Clouder and Sellers, 2004), and to positively influence staff recruitment, retention, support and development (Mullarkey, Keeley and Playle, 2001). Similarly, mentorship has been seen to benefit the integration of new graduates, to improve staff satisfaction and to improve staff retention (Carroll, 2004; Rosser et al., 2004; Smith et al., 2001; Tourigny and Pulich, 2005). Clearly, mentorship and clinical supervision have broadly similar goals, although, as described in the literature, mentorship tends to be more task-oriented and focused towards developing the professional abilities of more junior staff.

■ Research into mentorship and clinical supervision

Despite wide-ranging (and sometimes extravagant) expectations and claims, there is a limited literature detailing the outcomes of research into the effectiveness of mentoring and clinical supervision programmes. Of relevance to the Australian setting is the monograph published by Winstanley and White (2002) outlining models, measures and best practice in clinical supervision. These authors reviewed current evidence and recommended that the effectiveness of clinical supervision would be increased if it were held away from the workplace; occurred at least monthly; lasted for at least 60 minutes; and if supervisees were able to choose their supervisors. It was also suggested that group supervision may be more effective (Winstanley and White, 2002).

The literature reporting research into group mentoring and clinical supervision programmes is very limited, with few studies addressing the use of such programmes in mental health nursing. McCloughen and O'Brien (2005) have recently reported on the development of a mentorship programme for new graduates in mental health services in New South Wales in which new graduates were paired with an experienced mentor.

The apparent overlap (and associated confusions) between mentorship and clinical supervision and the lack of a definitive literature describing best practice pointed to the use of participatory action research methods for the project. The aim was to conduct a research project in which new graduates and clinical nurse consultants could work collaboratively to identify problems and solutions associated with transition into the workforce. The process of designing the programme was also informed by recommendations from the literature pointing to the importance of adequate preparation for mentors and supervisors (Rosser et al., 2004).

■ Materials and Methods

The broad aim of the project was to evaluate a group mentorship programme for new graduate nurses working in a public mental health service in one region of New South Wales. The project was designed to address the following research questions:

1. In what ways do new graduate nurses use group mentorship to manage the transition into the mental health workforce?

2. In what ways do clinical mentors use group mentorship to support new graduate nurses' transition into the mental health workforce?
3. What is the impact of group mentorship on the clinical practice of new graduate nurses working in mental health services?
4. What is the impact of group mentorship on new graduate nurses' decisions to remain in or leave employment in the mental health services?

A qualitative approach was adopted for the project, drawing on the methods of participatory action research (PAR). Participatory action research is a form of 'emic' (i.e. 'insider') research in which participants (in this case new graduate nurses and their clinical nurse consultant mentors) research their own professional actions. Action research originated in the early 20th century in the work of Kurt Lewin (1948), who studied how people learn to solve their own problems through self-education. In the decades since, action research has developed into a qualitative research methodology and has been adopted in the study of change in fields such as education (Elliot, 1991) and health care (Koch and Kralik, 2006).The approach of action research requires action as part of the research process itself and is focused on the researcher's professional values rather than methodological considerations (Street, 2003). Accordingly, the focus combines the collection of evidence to better understand a situation and collaborative action to improve it.

The approach taken is *situational* (i.e. addresses specific needs in context), *participatory* (i.e. involves those who are interested in, or will be affected by the outcome), and *self-evaluative* (i.e. enables self-evaluation of contribution to and functioning of the research activity) (Street, 2003). Action research thus provides an appropriate method for evaluating a group mentorship programme for new graduate nurses working in mental health services.

This evaluation study received ethics approval from the relevant university and area health human research ethics committees. The mentorship programme was implemented on two sites, with participants electing to join a mentorship group depending on their place of residence and work locations throughout the new graduate year. Participants were consenting new graduate nurses and experienced mental health nurses (i.e. clinical nurse consultants) working in the target mental health service. Three PAR groups consisting of (in total) 18 new graduate nurses and 5 clinical nurse consultant mentors were involved in the study. Following initial introductory workshops, each group met fortnightly for six months and then monthly for a further six months (one group met fortnightly for the second six-month period). Two PAR Groups commenced in July and August 2005. The third group commenced in February 2006. All three groups met regularly for twelve months.

Data collection for the project involved audiotape-recorded discussions within the groups, participative observation by research team members, and brief (one-to-two-page) summaries of discussions within the groups as recorded by the new graduates and/or the mentors. In the weeks between each meeting, data from the previous meeting was subjected to examination and analysis by research team members and returned to the groups in the form of a one-to-two-page summary of the previous meeting. Over time data from the audiotaped discussions, participative observations, participants' discussion summaries and research team members' meeting summaries became part of the research record for the project. While formal data collection instruments and interview schedules were not used in the study, at the commencement of each meeting participants were invited to review the main points that emerged from the previous meeting, to identify significant issues, concerns and possible solutions. Throughout the meetings, participant reflection was facilitated through the use of open-ended prompts such as 'What is significant for you in all of this?'

■ Results

□ Learning to fit in

Whilst the project generated a large amount of data, analysis indicated that much of this related to a relatively small number of themes. Foremost among these was 'learning to fit in', which highlighted the extent to which new graduates often experienced their work as taking place in a difficult and sometimes even hostile environment. The following excerpt from one of the new graduate participants provides an extreme example of the types of difficult situations new graduates could find themselves drawn into:

Group 1
    M/NG1[1]: I was the meat in the sandwich up there the other day....
    there was a yelling match between two staff members and then a third
    staff member came on the scene and started yelling, then they were
    asking my opinion of the whole thing; you know pretty well asked me
    who's side was I on ... It was in the courtyard in front of all the patients
    and then [the Nurse Unit Manager] came out and tried to diffuse the
    situation ... I had to give a statement the following day because it got
    that bad by the end of the shift, they were nearly at blows with each
    other.

---

[1] Participant interview excerpts have been coded to indicate gender (M = male; F = female), designation (NG = new graduate; CNC = Clinical Nurse Consultant) and differentiation (NG1 = new graduate 1; CNC2 = Clinical Nurse Consultant 2). Thus M/CNC1 = male Clinical Nurse Consultant 1 and F/NG3 = female new graduate 3.

While new graduates felt that many of their more experienced nursing colleagues were welcoming and supportive, others seemed disinterested or even hostile:

Group 3

F/NG1: I think there is an expectation that we have come out of Uni and we are RN's now right, and you go on the ward and a simple thing like transferring a [phone] call ... well how do I transfer the call? You don't know how to transfer a call? And [I] said no but if you show me then [I will] know. Or do an admission ... well can you show me ... I said I recognise the form from Uni but have never used it ... In the end you don't want to ask questions ... You know it is like who are you? I am a new grad, I want to them to know that. I am trying to fit in ...

What it was like to work alongside 'difficult staff' was a topic often raised in the mentorship groups. In some instances this could mean having to work with nurses who were uncaring and unmotivated in their approach to working with consumers:

Group 2

F/NG1: The people that intimidated me, they intimidate their patients on a worse level ...

Participants identified and discussed numerous examples of poor practice on the part of more senior nursing colleagues. Sometimes these examples related to an apparent lack of interest, knowledge and skills:

Group 3

F/NG1: ... we had a girl [admitted] ... She was absolutely paranoid about everything, all the patients, the staff, but I made a connection with her ... I sat down with her and she told me all this stuff and I am new. I went back to the staff ... and they said all right off you go [home]. I [said] I have just spoken to this girl because no one else would talk to her ... I want to tell you ... what she told me. That is going to affect her treatment ... that is how they related to her ... nobody is interested.

On other occasions the practices being discussed were ethically questionable:

Group 2

F/NG1: What fascinates me is that when you have a client who has schizophrenia but they are very quiet, no trouble ... They get their own room, they can have PRN twice a day; but if [they] are a bit noisy [they] are drug seeking; when [they] ask for PRN...a bit demanding; or if [they] ask for something [they] don't get their own room.

F/NG2: So it really comes down to how the staff member feels...don't bother me, I am there to be left alone because you really don't need that [PRN medication]; you are just pretending, [trying] to get at me.

For many of the new graduate participants the realisation that the knowledge and skills of many of the staff who had worked in mental health nursing for many years was at a relatively low level came as an unexpected surprise.

How best to deal with instances of observed poor practice by more experienced colleagues was clearly a major concern for participants. On the one hand, there was a strong sense of disquiet (and occasionally outrage) regarding what had been observed; one the other hand, there was a concern regarding what ought to be done in such circumstances. There was a feeling that any action taken by a new graduate would be unlikely to be taken seriously; there was also the possibility that the new graduate might be denigrated or even 'bullied' by more experienced staff:

Group 3

F/NG1: [The other day I was told I was to do the morning handover], I said, but I have never done one and this particular [experienced] nurse didn't want to do it. I said look, I don't mind coming in and watching...and then I will do it [next time]. He kept putting me one the spot...and the next day I [was off sick]. You know, the next day I got back he said to me: oh was that a mental health day or was that a sickie (i.e. a day of sick leave)...He said: couldn't [you] handle the workload?

A number of participants made the point that just being a new graduate was sufficient for them to be denigrated by some of the more experienced staff. Numerous examples were provided in all three PAR groups of the ways in which new comers (i.e. new graduates) could be 'kept in their place' by those who had worked in the service for some time. This might take the form of local resistance to new graduates being involved in the group mentorship programme. For instance, some participants were made to feel they would be leaving the ward short-staffed by attending the mentorship programme. This was despite the programme having the full support of the service executive and project funds having been made available to all participating clinical service areas to enable new graduates to be involved in mentorship programme meetings. Sometimes the pressure to conform to the expectations of colleagues in a particular clinical area was so great that the decision was made to not attend a meeting:

Group 1

> F/CNC1: So, really, being released [to attend the mentorship group] has been an ongoing issue for both of you...
>
> M/NG1: Not only that, I mean I have missed some weeks because I felt I probably shouldn't leave [the ward].
>
> F/NG2: Being able to go but just the guilt of you know [leaving the ward when things were busy].

How to deal with such pressures was often taken up with the mentors helping the new graduate participants to explore possible options in the action planning arising from the programme.

A number of participants were also concerned with the issue of how to manage staff who were habitually obstructive at work. While participants only came into contact with such staff occasionally, such experiences were clearly bewildering:

Group 1

> F/NG2: When you [were doing orientation to the ward] did someone go around with you and tick that off and say this is this?
>
> F/NG3: No, they just gave [the orientation check list] to me, if I had a problem I could go to them... But it is like they go, you are new and I don't want anything to do with you because you are new, because you don't know anything you can't help them so, they don't want to know you.
>
> F/NG2: I actually said to one of the more experienced nurses: don't you remember how that felt [being caught up in a medical emergency for] the first time, and she said: no, I can't remember...

☐ Negotiating organisational culture

Closely associated with the theme of fitting in was learning to negotiate the various nuances of the local health care organisational culture. This was often experienced as a tentative and grinding process of trial and error or working out the often unwritten protocols for working with more senior and experienced nursing colleagues:

Group 2

> NGM1: You hear stories filtering back about [a particular mental health unit]; it's a pretty hard place to work.
>
> NGF1: I really like it.
>
> NGM2: It's not hard, its how do I put it, there [are] a lot of established staff there and they have got their own little jokes and everything and it's just trying to figure out where it is appropriate to put a little witty aside and when to just stay out of it. All that sort of stuff... The unit

has been around for a while [and] staff that have worked there for a while ...

While some staff were welcoming and supportive others were much less so, and this could change from one shift to the next, or from one clinical location to another. For most participants the starting point was to determine who did what, both in formal and in informal terms. Clearly the influence exercised by some staff was based on holding a formal position in the organisation, such as a nurse manager or a clinical nurse consultant. In other cases, however, duration of employment, familiarity with the clinical setting, or the patients, or even strength of personality seemed to be the basis for a kind of informal power exercised by a particular staff member. In addressing concerns such as these participants spoke of working out the local staff 'politics', implying that unequal power relations were at work here and those with the greatest influence were not always staff holding formal positions within the organisation. One female new graduate, for instance, spoke of being openly challenged by a more experienced male counterpart to join those among the other staff who opposed the new models of care being developed and implemented throughout mental health services:

Group 2
F/NG2: I had one guy (i.e. an experienced registered nurse) come over to me and said: have you come over to the 'dark side' yet?
M/CNC1: He actually said that?
F/NG2: Yes, [I said] I am too positive. [He said] you will change.
M/CNC1: I think the 'dark side' is so seductive because you can be cynical, you can be lazy, you can see every patient as a waste of space ... but it is like you have to sell your soul for it.

Negotiating the local organisational culture could mean different things depending on the nature of the services within which new graduates were working. In acute services, familiarising oneself with and becoming comfortable using risk alerts was an important concern, and was closely related to 'specialling' and other aspects of getting along in a 'locked' environment. Another important concern was learning to be 'in charge', which often required working with less-qualified staff, many of whom were both influential and had far more experience working in mental health services.

Another key concern for new graduates was becoming accepted within the clinical team; this often involved being seen to have 'pitched in', or shadowing an experienced colleague through several hours of work:

Group 3
F/NG4: Being so new on the ward anyway I find that I tend to latch onto people that are open and friendly ... I just get a feeling that we are

going to get along. But I don't always get to work with those people and then I am a bit lost... because I don't know where to go...

The other side of this concern was the feeling that one had not been accepted. A range of negative emotions and experiences were associated with this, including feeling 'dumb' if it was implied or suggested that one lacked the knowledge and skills necessary for mental health nursing, or not knowing what to do in specific situations, or occasionally feeling as if one had deliberately been 'left in the dark', or had been set up to expose some form of shortcoming or failure. These concerns were well summarised by one of the (Group 3) mentors, paraphrasing comments made by a number of the new graduate participants: 'there is a culture of almost enjoying watching people struggle a little bit and perverse as that is to me, I think that is the reality'.

In another group, one of the participants described feeling foolish and powerless when he realised that the mental health nurse who had been assigned as his 'mentor' had continuously reported his 'inadequacies' to senior clinical staff. Some participants described being involved in complex games surrounding acceptance by more experienced colleagues. Other concerns involved complaints made against staff, or communication issues arising between nurses and medical staff.

Given the experiences described above, it is perhaps not surprising that learning to look after oneself at work is a recurring theme in the mentorship groups. This could include knowing when it might not be in one's best interests to agree to work overtime; feeling comfortable about declining a request to work overtime; managing fatigue, especially in the early months after commencing full-time employment; and ongoing concerns regarding whether one felt sufficiently competent to deal with the range of situations encountered at work. Such concerns also involved an element of adjusting to working life, which for most participants meant finding an effective balance between the demands of working life and those of social life.

☐ Developing 'know-how'

Despite the challenges associated with learning to 'fit in', new graduates clearly placed great importance on and worked hard to develop the 'know-how' necessary to provide effective mental health care. For the majority of new graduate participants the requirements for working effectively included *managing difficult clinical situations, being with consumers, being ethical*, and *becoming a skilled helper*. When participants discussed difficult clinical situations it was often in the context of consumers who were seen to pose an actual or potential threat to themselves (e.g. consumers considered to be at risk of self-injurious behaviour, posing a suicide threat or an absconding risk) or to others (e.g. consumers exhibiting aggressive, agitated or threatening behaviour).

However, there could also be concern for the comfort and dignity of those who might be compromised through clinical problems such as incontinence or reduced motivation. When new graduates discussed being with consumers this was usually in the context of wanting to develop the capacity for being therapeutically effective and involved recognition that engaging a consumer in a helping intervention necessitated the establishment and maintenance of therapeutic alliance. However, while recognising the importance of building a trusting relationship with a consumer, they often seemed unsure of just how one might go about developing the necessary skills to do so. Worryingly, they also seemed to have had little exposure to experienced mental health nurses who could model what was required. Sadly, it seemed that most of what participants had observed in more experienced mental health nursing colleagues interacting with those in their care were instances of consumers being dismissed, talked down to, or ignored by nurses:

Group 2
> F/NG1: [The] patient wants to use the phone, you have had a call today; oh but I have got this problem; you have had a call. [And the patient is told to] go away! It is rude and it is disrespectful and the patient has nowhere to go.

Alongside this desire to build the technical capacity required to manage clinical situations effectively was a concern to develop ethical know-how; that is, to be able to work with consumers and health professional colleagues in an ethical manner. To this end, discussions ranged over topics such as what ought to be done when it was felt a consumer had been demonised by staff – for instance, working with a person with a history of child abuse, or working with someone diagnosed with borderline personality disorder. In particular, participants sought guidance regarding how such situations might be managed should they wish to take a contrary stand to the prevailing views of staff. Another, widely discussed concern was what was seen as the apparent misuse of 'duty of care', where the notion might be enlisted as part of the rationale to place inappropriate restrictions on a consumer:

Group 1
> F/NG1: I have heard duty of care bounced around a lot for actually the reason we persist against what a patient wants. Have you heard it much?
> M/N1: You get that thrown around down there [i.e. a particular ward] a bit.
> F/NG1: So what does it mean? When it is heard in context?

M/NG1: They feel you know they need to be showered to make them comfortable and hygienic.

F/NG2: It seems to be the way they get [the patients] to do things [they] really don't want to do.

M/NG1: A manipulation tactic.

Along similar lines:

Group 1

F/NG1: Sometimes you don't pre-warn them [the patients] like you know the outcome, you know what is going to happen.

F/CNC2: I think you should always pre-warn clients.

F/NG1: Well, when this [patient] she thought she was going to get out [of hospital] and we weren't allowed to say that we were going in for a two-month order to keep you in here, we weren't allowed to tell her that.

F/CNC2: Who made that decision?

F/NG1: [The NUM], but we weren't allowed to say you are going to be here for two months. I wished her luck and hoped she got what she wanted all the time knowing that she was going to have a two-month stay. That's really hard but I wasn't in the position to do that...

Another topic raised by participants was the strategic use of self-disclosure; under what circumstances this may or may not be appropriate. Other topics raised in this area included the withholding of information from consumers, or circumstances in which it appeared that punishment was being administered in the guise of treatment.

It was also noteworthy that even at this early stage in their careers as registered nurses, participants were already interested in finding out about options for developing more advanced clinical skills, such as cognitive behaviour therapy, dialectical behaviour therapy and motivational interviewing.

■ Discussion

McCloughen and O'Brien (2006) have recently described the problems associated with implementing inter-agency collaborative research projects such as mentorship programmes designed to support new graduate nurses entering the mental health workforce. They outline a number of problems including communication, environmental factors, politics and power relations and organisational culture that contributed to the demise of the project described in their fascinating article.

In many ways our experience was similar to that that described by McCloughen and O'Brien (2006), and yet our project was successfully conducted within the anticipated timeframe, and has subsequently informed decision-making regarding arrangements for the provision of structured support for new graduates in the mental health service in question. To some extent we would attribute the success of our project down to our having anticipated and planned for the types of problems described by McCloughen and O'Brien (2006). For instance, we sought to consult widely with all identified stakeholders and in particular worked closely with (and had the strong support of) the executive management of the service and we engaged clinical leaders to undertake the mentorship role.

Nonetheless, despite several letters being sent to managers pointing out the availability of funding to release new graduates from clinical areas to attend mentorship groups and explaining the process for claiming such funds, problems were experienced throughout the life of the project in releasing some new graduates from some clinical areas. Indeed, by the end of the project a substantial proportion of the project funds set aside for the release of participants to attend groups had not been claimed – this was unexpected. A recurring theme throughout the period of data collection was the extent to which new graduates experienced constant questioning of the usefulness of the project, or were exposed to criticism from colleagues that they were leaving to attend the group when the service was short-staffed, or operating at full capacity. It is perhaps not surprising that under these circumstances a number of participants reported feeling guilty about attending the mentorship groups.

We should not underestimate the impact of stigma on staff working in mental health services and the ways this may affect decisions to remain in or leave this area of health care work. A recent study (Wigney and Parker, 2007) of medical students' concerns regarding a career in psychiatry raised similar issues to those discussed by participants in this study. In particular, medical students painted a picture of (public sector) psychiatry as an area of medical practice characterised by low prestige, limited treatments and difficult patients. Similar 'stigmatising perspectives' are almost certainly at work in nursing.

There is clearly a great need for high-quality, positive educational experiences in mental health service in undergraduate nursing curricula. However, we need to question the often-found emphasis on 'challenging patients' that has undergraduate students thinking about the risks associated with nursing people with disorders such as schizophrenia, or borderline personality disorder, before they have had a chance to develop mental health literacy (Jorm, 2000; Jorm et al., 2006). Having established a more positive inclination towards mental health nursing among undergraduates, we could then follow this up in the graduate year by having new graduates work closely with the most clinically skilled nurses in a service, who could provide structured forms of mentorship. In the Australia context, this would ordinarily be clinical nurse specialists and clinical nurse consultants.

At least equal consideration needs to be given to attracting and retaining new graduates – our most precious resource, within the mental health workforce, with workforce development initiatives being an important aspect of strategies for staff retention and service improvement.

It is here that mentorship programmes can have a significant impact. Whether this happens or not will depend on the degree of influence that can be exercised by the profession, and the priority that health planners and service managers give to developing the mental health nursing workforce in the coming years. While recruitment, retention and workforce development continue to be afforded low strategic priority (and thus inadequate resources), the current problems are likely to remain, or become even more severe. The new graduate nurses involved in this project were resourceful, creative registered nurses who needed support – when they received it they thrived; when they didn't they struggled. Mostly they thrived.

■ Conclusion

Like many other health and social care professionals, new graduate nurses working in a regional mental health service experience their graduate year as a process of learning to 'fit in' to what often seems like a hostile working environment. While working with more senior nursing staff, some of whom seem unmotivated and/or hostile, new graduates also find themselves negotiating the health care organisational culture. At the same time they work hard to develop the 'know-how' necessary to work effectively in mental health services – including 'being with consumers', 'being ethical', and 'becoming a skilled helper'. Consolidating initial employment and career planning are also key concerns. The emphasis on 'learning to fit in' sometimes undermines opportunities to mobilise the idealism brought from university studies as a progressive force to bring local improvements to mental health care. Group mentorship by expert mental health nurses provide support to enable the new graduates to make a difference.

References

Australian Health Workforce Advisory Committee (2003). Australian mental health nursing supply, recruitment and retention. *Australian Health Report 2003*. Sydney: Australian health Workforce Advisory Committee.
Berg, A. and Hallberg, I. R. (2000). The meaning and significance of clinical group supervision and supervised individually planned nursing care as narrated by nurses on a general team psychiatric ward. *Australian and New Zealand Journal of Mental Health Nursing*, 9 (3): 110–127.

Carroll, K. (2004). Mentoring: A human becoming perspective. *Nursing Science Quarterly*, 17 (4): 318–322.

Clare, J., Edwards, H., Brown, D. and White, J. (2003). Evaluating clinical learning environments: Creating education–practice partnerships and clinical education benchmarks for nursing. *Learning Outcomes and Curriculum Development in Major Disciplines: Nursing Phase 2 Final Report*, School of Nursing and Midwifery, Flinders University, Adelaide.

Clinton, M. and Hazelton, M. (2001a). Scoping mental health nursing education. *Australian and New Zealand Journal of Mental Health Nursing*, 9 (1): 2–10.

Clinton, M. and Hazelton, M. (2001b). Scoping the Australian mental health nursing workforce. *Australian and New Zealand Journal of Mental Health Nursing*, 9 (2): 56–64.

Clinton, M. and Hazelton, M. (2001c). Scoping practice issues in the Australian mental health nursing workforce. *Australian and New Zealand Journal of Mental Health Nursing*, 9 (3): 100–109.

Clinton, M. and Hazelton, M. (2001d). Scoping the prospects of Australian mental health nursing. *Australian and New Zealand Journal of Mental Health Nursing*, 9 (4): 159–165.

Clinton, M. and Hazelton, M. (2002). Towards a foucauldian reading of the Australian mental health nursing workforce. *International Journal of Mental Health Nursing*, 1 (11): 18–23.

Clinton, M., du Boulay, S., Hazelton, M. and Horner, B. (2001). Mental health nursing education and the health labour force: A literature review. *National Review of Nurse Education*. www.dest.gov.au/highered/programmes/nursing, Canberra.

Clouder, L. and Sellers, J. (2004). Reflective practice and clinical supervision: An interprofessional perspective. *Journal of Advanced Nursing*, 46 (3): 262–269.

Cobal, A. (1998). Graduate nurses: Exploring the transition from student to registered nurse. Unpublished Honours thesis, La Trobe University.

Commonwealth of Australia (2002). *National Review of Nurse Education 2002. Our Duty of Care*. Canberra: AGPS.

Elliot, J. (1991). *Action Research for Educational Change*. Buckingham: Open University Press.

Farrell, G. and Carr, J. (1996). Who cares for the mentally ill? Theory and practice hours with a 'mental illness' focus in nursing curricula in Australian universities. *Australian and New Zealand Journal of Mental Health Nursing*, 5: 77–83.

Gabbard, G. (1997). Lessons to be learned from the study of sexual boundary violations. *Australian and New Zealand Journal of Psychiatry*, 31: 321–327.

Holmes, C. (2006). The slow death of psychiatric nursing: What next? *Journal of Psychiatric and Mental Health Nursing*, 13: 401–415.

Jorm, A. F. (2000). Mental health literacy: Public knowledge about mental disorders. *British Journal of Psychiatry*, 177: 396–401.

Jorm, A. F., Barney, L. J., Christensen, H., Highet, N. J., Kelly, C. M. and Kitchener, B. A. (2006). Research into mental health literacy: What we know and what we still need to know. *Australian and New Zealand Journal of Psychiatry*, 40: 3–5.

Kilstoff, K. and Rochester, S. (2003). Hit the floor running: Transitional experiences of graduates previously trained as enrolled nurses. *Australian Journal of Advanced Nursing*, 22 (1): 13–17.

Koch, T. and Kralik, D. (2006). *Participatory Action Research in Health Care*. Carlton: Blackwell Publishing.

Kramer, M. (1974). *Reality Shock: Why Nurses Leave Nursing*. Mosby. St Louis Missouri.

Lewin, K. (1948). *Resolving Social Conflicts*. New York: Harper.

Lindahl, B. and Norberg, A. (2002). Clinical group supervision in an intensive care unit: A space for relief, and for sharing emotions and experiences of care. *Journal of Clinical Nursing*, 11 (6): 809–818.

McCloughen, A. and O'Brien, L. (2005). Development of a mentorship programme for new graduate nurses in mental health. *International Journal of Mental Health Nursing*, 14 (4): 276–284.

McCloughen, A. and O'Brien, L. (2006). Interagency collaborative research projects: Illustrating potential problems and finding solutions in the nursing literature. *International Journal of Mental Health Nursing*, 15 (3): 171–180.

Mental Health Nurse Education Taskforce (2008). Final report: Mental health in pre-registration nursing courses. *Mental health Workforce Advisory Committee, Department of Human Services*, Victoria.

Moorhouse, C. (1992). *Registered Nurse. The First Year of Professional Practice*. Melbourne: La Trobe University Press.

Mullarkey, K., Keeley, P. and Playle, J. F. (2001). Multiprofessional clinical supervision: Challenges for mental health nurses. *Journal of Psychiatric and Mental Health Nursing*, 8 (3): 205–211.

Rosser, M., Rice, A. M., Campbell, H. and Jack, C. (2004). Evaluation of a mentorship programme for specialist practitioners. *Nurse Education Today*, 24 (8): 596–604.

Smith, L. S., McAllister, L. E. and Crawford, C. S. (2001). Mentoring benefits and issues for public health nurses. *Public Health Nursing*, 18 (2): 101–107.

Street, A. (2003). Action research. In: D. Schneider et al. (eds.) *Nursing Research: Methods, Critical Appraisal and Utilisation* (2nd ed.). pp. 219–231.

Tourigny, L. P. and Pulich, M. P. (2005). A critical examination of formal and informal mentoring among nurses. *Health Care Manager January/March*, 24 (1): 68–76.

Wigney, T. and Parker, G. (2007). Medical student observations on a career in psychiatry. *Australian and New Zealand Journal of Psychiatry*, 41 (9): 726–731.

Winstanley, J., and White, E. (2002). Clinical supervision: Models measures and best practice. *Nurse Researcher*, 10 (4): 7–38.

End Note: Thoughts in search of a thinker

Tony Warne and Sue McAndrew

As this book draws to a close we hope that for the reader it has been thought-provoking, with the aim of this last chapter being to pull together the central issues that have emerged throughout the book so that we can think more creatively in how we approach and facilitate the learning of health and social care professionals. Our starting point in this final chapter is the familiar concept that suggests that effective learning is where the individual is enabled to gain insight from within self by seeing for themselves the whole pattern of what they are learning. The individual experience here is an important constituent of our thinking.

For example, creativity is sometimes deemed to be an aspect of organisational and institutional policy. However, in this situation, the measures put in place to foster creativity – that is imagination, thought, thinking, personal growth and criticality – produce an environment whereby aspiration is routinely not realised. Institutionally and individually such approaches displace the 'matrix of the mind' (Ogden, 1986), an environment grounded in healthy dialectical relationships (inter- and intra-subjectively), thus damaging creative 'potential space' (Winnicott, 1971). For educationalists it is as much a matter of creating 'spaces' to think as it is about taking 'time' to think (Wittgenstein, 1980, p. 28). However, in Chapter 1 Peter Morrall warns of how 'Western universities murder thinking.' Thus it is not the teacher who 'passes on' their insight to the learner, but who facilitates learning experiences through which the learner gains insight for themselves. As Margaret McAllister suggests in Chapter 11, this will require moving from a transmission model of teaching to a transformative model that emphasises transaction. An important theme running through the book has been how such intra- and inter-subjectivity can be achieved through the various types of creative learning opportunities described in many of the chapters (in particular see Part 2).

Learning is an individual dynamic process whereby connections are constantly changing and their structure reformatted (Cross, 1991). Students construct their own meaning by talking, listening, writing, reading and reflecting on content, ideas, issues and concerns (Meyers and Jones, 1993). Creativity depends upon an intimate, flexible and dynamic time/space for thinking. It requires a new way of thinking about the traditional roles and characteristics of the academy. This is an approach that can be difficult to effect. As we saw in the early chapters, often the narrative of organisational processes in contemporary universities defines the parameters of the spaces for thinking and learning. This organisational paradigm often fails to support the dialogic relationships which promote creative developmental thinking, a process intrinsic and fundamental to ensuring creative approaches to learning in universities. In Chapter 13, Dawn Freshwater and Philip Esterhuizen draw our attention to the work of Bruner (1996), who believed 'thinking about thinking to be the principle ingredient of any empowering practice of education'.

Contemporary institutions' explicit preoccupation with assuring, monitoring and managing creative dialogue can prevent creative processes, and will often result in institutional battles that disadvantage the teacher and student (Power, 1997; Warne, 2007). Through rituals of verification institutional and governmental emphases both subtly and, on some occasions, spectacularly damage the university as a creative space (Mac Rury, 2007). Consider, for example, the polarised and hotly contested debates around the relative merits and importance of teaching and research (Thompson and Watson, 2006), where emphasis and support is often given to one and not the other in what should be an integrated approach to learning (see Chapter 12).

Throughout this book, recognition is given to the importance of research as one aspect of producing the evidence for learning, contemplation and reflection. The approach has been to develop a conceptual approach that moves beyond the simple polarised notions of research and teaching or theory and practice. Brew (2006) has described this more integrated view of the work of universities as being that of 'inclusive scholarly knowledge-building communities of practice' (p. 180). She argues, following Barnett (2000), that university teaching and learning should be aimed above all else at preparing students for a world which is uncertain, super complex and unpredictable. Indeed, in Chapter 2 Gary Rolfe urges that innovative curricula and learning interventions must occur in conjunction with the equally important epistemological project of innovative research and practice development. Warne and McAndrew (2007) have described this process of preparation as that which should be enabling individuals (teachers, practitioners and students) to stay at the edge between knowing and not knowing. In closing this book, this End Note sets out to explore these notions more fully. Perhaps given our background, it is unsurprising that we chose to draw upon the work of Bion, teacher, psychoanalyst and person, to set the scene for this exploration.

■ Harnessing thoughts

Bion argued that 'the mind grows through exposure to truth' (Bion, 1962). This growth (of mind) is related to the ability of the individual to act more consistently and rigorously in relation to truth (Symington and Symington, 1996). Arguably this is not something that is likely to occur where the prime concern is to ensure that a predetermined curriculum has been 'covered'.

We are persuaded, and as we have tried to demonstrate in this book, our approach to students is not predicated on the notion of students being empty vessels waiting to be filled, but are individuals who arrive at the institution with their own perceptual framework, encompassing personal experiences, imagination and thought. This would suggest that students arrive with a multitude of thoughts that are awaiting a thinker, conveying a picture of infinite potential thoughts available to the mind engaged in learning from experience (Symington and Symington, 1996). To learn from experience there has to be an awareness of the emotional experience. Such awareness prompts thoughts, existing prior to their realisation. Thinking is the capacity to think the thoughts which already exist (Bion, 1962). The essence of thinking encapsulates both the intra- and inter-personally dialogic, requiring and enabling meaningful movement between the subjective experience and external knowledge. In Chapter 11, Margaret McAllister talks of the 'language of possibility' needing to be practised if ideas for the future are to emerge. In harnessing past and present individual experiences and facilitating 'thought full' thinking health and social care students will be offered the opportunity to make sense of available theories and the experiences of other, thus arriving at a 'truth'.

It is in our contemplation of Bion's work that we, like others, (French and Simpson, 1999) see the effects of exposure to this truth as a learning which comes from working at the edge between knowing and not knowing. French and Simpson (1999) note that this implies two necessary elements for effective work: firstly, an appropriate level of knowledge; and secondly, being disposed to engage with not knowing. They argue that often we are all prepared to work at this edge. This is when the necessary combination of knowledge and disposition is shared and an empathic, helping and supportive relationship approach exists (Rogers, 1969). Unfortunately, as teachers or health and social care practitioners, we are often expected to do this work on behalf of others because we are 'the ones who know'.

■ Knowledge, knowing and the space between – not knowing

As we have seen in the opening chapters of this book, knowledge can be both explicit and tacit. Explicit knowledge can be captured and written down in documents or databases. Examples of explicit knowledge include instruction manuals, written procedures, best practices, lessons learned and research findings. Explicit knowledge is systematic and easily communicated in the form of hard data or codified procedures. It can be articulated in formal language and can easily be transmitted across individuals. Hence theoretical knowledge is part of explicit knowledge.

Tacit knowledge is not available as a text and may conveniently be regarded as 'silent knowledge', an understanding in a given context without being stated, or 'knowing'. It involves intangible factors embedded in personal beliefs, experiences and values, and comprises experience and an application of explicit knowledge that resides only with the individual. Tacit knowledge can be difficult to access (see Chapter 9 for one approach to access such knowledge) as it is often not known to others; indeed, most people are not aware of the knowledge they themselves possess or of its value to others. Tacit knowledge is valuable because it provides context for people, places, ideas and experiences. It generally requires extensive personal contact and trust to be shared effectively or even recognised as valued knowledge.

While tacit knowledge can be possessed by itself, explicit knowledge must rely on being tacitly understood and applied, hence all knowledge is either tacit or rooted in tacit knowledge. By paying attention to the tacit dimension we can begin to make sense of the place of intuition and hunches in informal education practice and how we can come to a better understanding of what might be going on in different situations.

Arguably, theoretical knowledge may act as a hindrance to the processes of 'knowing', in that we may become distracted from what we are experiencing, rather than learning from what is occurring in the here–and-now relationships (Reeder, 2002). Such knowing requires the development of a high level of insightfulness and under-standing of the various manifestations of the 'professional and personal self', a type of 'knowing' that is not readily available to many. In this instance, knowing refers to an unconscious primary process, a product of our history which encompasses our beliefs and values, and is culturally and socially bounded (Reeder, 2002). We suggest that often the development of such insightfulness and knowing is also inhib-ited by current educational processes of 'becoming' and 'being' a health or social care professional and, paradoxically, the rhetoric of student empowerment as medi-ated by some strands of managerialism in contemporary higher education (Freire, 1972). Such educational processes are often concerned with the emphasis on the development of a 'professional self', and one concerned with reinforcing profes-sional distance and boundaries (McQueen, 2000). This is an approach that fails to recognise the unconscious 'personal self' and the impact this 'self' has on the development of and engagement with others in everyday practice (see Marie Crow's Chapter 6 for the implications of this).

Theoretical knowledge can also provide a sanctuary for the professional who unconsciously wishes to distance themselves from the emotional milieu of their patients, thus avoiding the personal consequences implicit in the emotional bur-den of caring (Warne and McAndrew, 2005). For example, nurses responding to the belief that they cannot effectively help the person if they become too involved in the individuals emotional distress develop and maintain a 'professional distance' in their nurse–patient relationships. Such 'professional distance' has also been described as the 'dependency distance' (Warne and McAndrew, 2004). However, in order to know the world of the person, it is necessary to find out what their expe-rience is at that particular time, and what sense and meaning they attach to that experience. Phil Barker and Poppy Buchanan-Barker (see Chapter 3) refer to this as 'storied lives' whereby sense can be made of complex concepts by discovering what the concepts mean to the individual storyteller. For us this requires learning to work at the edges of 'knowing and not knowing', a place that can initially feel uncomfortable because of the uncertainty it elicits within both lecturer and student.

■ Between knowing and not knowing

French and Simpson (1999) suggest that our best work happens when we don't know what we are doing. We argue that, likewise, practitioners, teachers and stu-dents engaged in health and social care education and practice might be more effective if they acknowledged and worked with the possibility that they do not know what is actually going on; even where they think they know what it was they intended to happen or what they think is occurring.

Acknowledging the possibility that they might not know the response to be taken in meeting patients' needs can facilitate remaining open to the dynamics of the present moment. Best evidence approaches to care and treatment are not always easily accommodated in the here-and-now encounter with the patient (see Chapters 2 and 12). Despite professional development claims of lifelong learning, many students and their various educators at times often have difficulty in creating opportunities for theory to be deconstructed, re-constructed and *fitted* to reflect the individual patient and their health needs (Warne et al., 2004). Thus when the use of best evidence approaches are transposed to the clinical situation, their effectiveness might be compromised by the patient's knowledge of self, even where this is not openly articulated. Where health and social care professionals are able to remain open to the dynamics of the encounter, their interventions are informed more by the sense-making and the knowing that might arise out of the interaction rather than on the basis of pre-constituted knowledge and thus predetermined practice. It is embracing this openness that capability begins to transcend competence. Competence is what we would expect from the health and social care practitioner trained to carry out a set of familiar tasks in prescribed ways and in familiar contexts, whereas capability is the ability to deal with unfamiliar demands and tasks in unfamiliar situations (Watson, 2006). Being able to create learning opportunities that promote effectiveness and capability in relation to dealing with the unexpected, unintended and troublesome can be a difficult task.

■ Troublesome knowledge

It is a difficult task for all those engaged in dealing with the uncertainty resulting from the abandonment of the familiar and previously known knowledge in the light of the integration of new and sometimes troublesome knowledge. Troublesome knowledge arises from the process of re-conceptualising how to make sense of another person's illness and deliver care in accordance with individual need, particularly where this differs from previous experiences. Not only will such a situation impact on the personal subjectivity of the individual, challenging their ontological security, it is likely to render them helpless and disempowered as a professional (Land, 2004). Locating oneself in such a position can be uncomfortable and lead to defensiveness, hostility and anxiety (Meyer and Land, 2003; Clouder, 2005). Existing certainties challenged in this way can lead to the student and teacher experiencing a lack of authenticity and/or their engagement in mimicry (Clouder, 2005). What students want is trouble-free knowledge (Land, 2004), which, given the messiness of practice within which students learn, is unlikely to occur (Warne and McAndrew, 2006). Likewise, what teachers want to give is clear explicit knowledge with which the student can start to learn to perform capably.

Caring in the professional context of health and social care has been described as complex and elusive (Paley, 2001). In preparing people to work within an increasingly turbulent health and social care arena the modern curriculum does not often lend itself to the emotional dimension of professional learning, through the explication of tacit knowledge. Exposing students to new and/or alternative ways of thinking and knowing will undoubtedly lead to uncertainty and for most will initially challenge them with troublesome knowledge (Meyer and Land, 2005). Benner and Wrubel (1989) argue that in a highly technical society that values individualism and competitiveness caring practices have always been fragile. Thus dealing with troublesome knowledge will require the student to undergo a transformation in their sense of identity as they engage with the multiplicity of discourses that underpin health and social care. Caring discourses are currently part of the implicit curriculum and we hope that by engaging with this book more attempts will be made to make them explicit (see also Chapters 5, 6, 8, 9, 10 and 11). The traditional caring discourse whereby emotion is considered to interfere with rational choice is now being challenged as it is recognised that in situations of indeterminacy emotions can be a useful source of knowledge in promoting decision-making (Johns, 2000).

■ Thoughts in search of a thinker

Teaching that focuses on skills and competencies that are categorised and criterion-referenced in a way that possibly lacks sensitivity to emphasise to the student the importance of their emotional self needs to be challenged. However, such qualities are more likely to be brought to fruition if those expected to portray such qualities are themselves in receipt of the same or similar qualities from the organisations – in this instance, educationalists – they are affiliated to. Indeed, in Chapter 13, Dawn Freshwater and Philip Esterhuizen challenge educationalists regarding the extent to which they allow the natural talents of students to emerge and how they support and nurture them to the point of gaining independence in their professional role. Sullivan (1953) described this as the need for reflective appraisal, a concept akin to mirroring. In relation to providing health and social care it is the 'emotional' component of the inter-subjective relationship that needs to be captured through the experience of mirroring.

Psychoanalytically, mirroring equates to how the original others view and respond to the child (Winnicott, 1971). The psychic need for mirroring and idealising self-object experiences form the rudimentary basis of a cohesive self. A cohesive sense of self lays the foundation for discovering one's existence as a temporal being capable of creating meaning. As the child grows and develops their sense of security, they are slowly able to let go of the a priori values conferred by the parents and move towards an understanding that values are created rather than given and always have the potential to change in the light of experience. Such experiences are present throughout our lives and, in developing and mediating meaning, values can be conceived which synergistically augment one's sense of meaning (Yalom, 1980).

Listening to students who wish to share their experiences and be given opportunity to explore and have their uncertainties legitimised will be helpful in moving students towards, and hopefully through, the threshold of their learning (Clouder, 2005). Teachers do not need to possess ready answers and it is good that students see this is the case and that many issues relating to health and social care are multivariate in their resolve.

Creative approaches to learning can promote opportunities to extend and link ordinary and extraordinary elements of experience, emotional knowing and knowledge. To facilitate such approaches universities need to foster and support environments and relationships where thinking capacity, developmental experience and productive transformation can thrive (Wittenburg et al., 1983). As educationalists we need to move our students towards the development of their own capacity to create potential space so that any resolution becomes not a matter of exchange, mutuality or reciprocity, but of an ongoing capacity to think, engage and act creatively in and around the space of the 'other'. In doing so, the emphasis is not on identity or mastery but on creativity and the potential it brings for understanding and meaning (Ogden, 1986). A good enough institution affords an optimisation of the ongoing engagement between the intimate subjective life of individuals and the work with(in) and between self and other. Good enough pedagogic relating and academic creativity grounded in and consistent with an understanding of human experience rooted optimally in positive dialogical relationships will promote personal transformations and a (re)emergence of capacities for thinking, reflexive practice and creative care.

References

Barnett, R. (2000). *Realizing the University: In an Age of Supercomplexity*. Buckingham: SRHE/Open University Press.

Benner, P. and Wrubel, J. (1989). *The Primary of Caring: Stress and Coping in Health and Illness*. Menlo Park: Addison-Wesley.

Bion, W. (1962). *Learning from Experience*. London: Heinemann.

Brew, A. (2006). *Research and Teaching: Beyond the Divide*. Basingstoke: Palgrave Macmillan.

Cross, K. P. (1991). College Teaching: What do we know about it? *Innovative Higher Education*, 16 (1), 7–25.

Bruner, J. (1996). *The Culture of Education*. London: Harvard University Press.

Clouder, L. (2005). Caring as a 'threshold' concept: transforming students in higher education into health(care) professionals. *Teaching in Higher Education*, 10(4), 505–517.

French, R. and Simpson, P. (1999). Our best work happens when we don't know what we are doing. *Socio-Analysis*, 1(2), 216–230.

Freire, P. (1972). *Pedogogy of the Oppressed*. London: Penguin.

Land, R. (2004). *Using Threshold Concepts to Identify Troublesome Knowledge: An Innovative Approach to Course Design*. Health and Social Sciences Teaching and Learning Conference, Coventry University.

MacRory, I. (2007). Institutional Creativity and Pathologies of Potential Space: The Modern University. Creativity or Conformity? Building Cultures of Creativity in Higher Education, a conference organised by the University of Wales Institute, Cardiff in collaboration with the Higher Education Academy.

Meyers, C. and Jones, T. B. (1993). *Promoting Active Learning: Strategies for the college classroom*. San Francisco: Jossey-Bass.

McQueen, A. (2000). Nurse-patient relationships and partnership in hospital care. *Journal of Clinical Nursing*, 9 (5), 723–731.

Meyer, J. H. F. and Land, R. (2005). Threshold concepts and troublesome knowledge (2): Epistemological considerations and a conceptual framework for teaching and learning. *Higher Education*, 49 (3), 373–388.

Ogden, T. (1986). *The Matrix of the Mind*. London: Karnac.

Paley, J. (2001). An archaeology of caring knowledge. *Journal of Advanced Nursing*, 36(2), 188–198

Power, M. (1997). *The Audit Society: Rituals of Verification*. Oxford: Oxford University Press.

Reeder, J. (2002). From knowledge to competence: Reflections on theoretical work. *International Journal of Psychoanalysis*. 83, 799–809.

Rogers, C. (1969). *Freedom to Learn*. Merrill New York.

Sullivan, H. S. (1953). *Interpersonal Relations Theory of Psychiatry*. NY: Norton and Norton.

Symington, J. and Symington, N. (1996). *The Clinical Thinking of Wilfred Bion*. London: Routledge.

Thompson, D. and Watson, R. (2006). Professors of nursing: What do they profess? *Nurse Education in Practice*, 6, 123–126.

Warne, T. (2007). *University Based Nurse Training and the Rituals of Verification: Devaluing Practice Based Evidence.* Invited Paper 7th International Nursing Conference, Comenius University, Martin, Slovakia.

Warne, T. and McAndrew, S. (2004). Nursing, nurse education and professionalisation in a contemporary context. In T. Warne and S. McAndrew (Eds.) *Using Patient Experience in Nurse Education.* Palgrave Publishers: London.

Warne, T. and McAndrew, S. (2005). The shackles of abuse: Unprepared to work at the edges of reason? *Journal of Psychiatric and Mental Health Nursing*, 12, 679–685.

Warne, T. and McAndrew, S. (2006). Splitting the difference: The heroes and villains of mental health policy and nursing practice. *Issues in Mental Health Nursing*, 27(9), 1001–1013.

Warne, T. and McAndrew, S. (2007). Passive Patient or Engaged Expert? Using a Ptolemaic approach to enhance Mental Health Nurse Education and Practice. *International Journal of Mental Health Nursing*, 16(4), 224–229.

Warne, T., McAndrew, S., Hepworth, H., Collins, E. and McGregor, S. (2004). Looking Back, Stepping Forward. In T. Warne and S. McAndrew (Eds). *Using Patient Experience in Nurse Education* Palgrave Publishers.

Watson, R. (2006). Is there a role for higher education in preparing nurses. *Nurse Education Today*, 26, 622–626.

Winnicott, D. (1971). *Playing and Reality.* New York: Basic Books.

Wittenstein, L. (1980). *Culture and Value.* Oxford: Blackwell.

Yalom, I. D. (1980). *Existential Psychotherapy.* USA: Basic Books.

Appendix: Films with a Health-Related Theme

Alcoholism – *Barfly 1989; When a Man Loves a Woman 1994*

Anxiety/Neurosis – *Analyse This 1999; Play it Again Sam 1972*

Attention Deficit Hyperactivity Disorder (ADHD) – *Thumbsucker 2005*

Bereavement – *Ordinary People 1980; Blessed 2004*

Bipolar Disorder – *Mr Jones 1993; The Flying Scotsman 2006*

Cancer – *Champions 1984; Ikiru 1952*

Cerebral Palsy – *My Left Foot 1989*

Child Health/Development – *About a Boy 2002*

Cystic Fibrosis – *Lifebreath 1997*

Dementia – *Away from Her 2006; Iris 2001; The Notebook 2004*

Depression – *The Hours 2002; Prozac Nation 2001*

Diabetes – *Panic Room 2002; Steel Magnolias 1989*

Disfigurement – *The Elephant Man 1980; Mask 1985*

Domestic Violence/Abuse – *The Prince of Tides 1991; The Color Purple 1985*

Drug Abuse – *Trainspotting 1996; The Man with the Golden Arm 1955; Christiane F 1981*

Eating Disorder – *For the Love of Nancy 1994; Hunger Point 2003*

Epilepsy – *First do no Harm 1997*

Heart Disease – *Paris 2008*

HIV/AIDS – *Touch Me 1997; Philadelphia 1993*

Learning Disability – *I Am Sam 2001; Rain Man 1988*

Obsessive Compulsive Disorder (OCD) – *As Good as It Gets 1997; The Aviator 2005; Matchstick Men 2003*

Physical Disability – *Born on the Fourth of July 1989; The Sea Inside 2004*

Schizophrenia – *A Beautiful Mind 2001; Shine 1996; Some Voices 2000*

Terminal Illness – *Terms of Endearment 1983; Love Story 1970*

Transplantation – *21 Grams 2003*

Tuberculosis – *Infinity 1996*

Index